WP B SMART /SERIES

BACK PAIN

Kusal Goonewardena

WP

Published by
Wilkinson Publishing Pty Ltd
ACN 006 042 173
Level 4, 2 Collins Street, Melbourne, Vic 3000
Tel: 03 9654 5446 www.wilkinsonpublishing.com

International distribution by Pineapple Media Ltd
(www.pineapple-media.com) ISSN 2203-2789
Copyright © 2014 Kusal Goonewardena

National Library of Australia Cataloguing-in-Publication entry:

Author: Goonewardena, Kusal, author.

Title: Back pain / Kusal Goonewardena.

ISBN: 9781922178787 (paperback)

Subjects: Backache--Treatment--Popular works.
                   Backache--Physical therapy--Popular works.

Dewey Number: Dewey Number: 617.564

Photos and illustrations by agreement with international agencies,
photographers and illustrators from iStockphoto.
Photos also by agreement with Rodney Stewart.

Design: Jo Hunt
Printed in China

AUTHOR INTRODUCTION

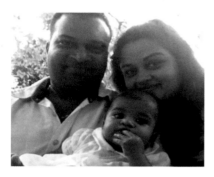

I have been on a journey that has allowed me to accumulate knowledge and understand how the body works. I have learnt that low back pain can be debilitating, frustrating and scary for those sufferers who cannot find a solution. Some have given up because they realise that they have done as much as they can within what their community healthcare services provide. This is not a limitation about them it is simply a limitation on the resources they have access to. I am here to tell you that the world is now readily accessible and no one should ever give up. There is always an answer out there. I hope this book spurs you on to keep finding solutions. We live in the age of technology, science and innovation, and these can come together to help people who suffer back pain. We have the potential to find new solutions every year.

I would love to hear your story of success, how and what you have done to overcome your pain, what road you have travelled, and continue to travel to find a solution. Keep in touch.

My email address is: kusal@elitekademy.com

Thank you for reading this and may your life be happy and joyous in every way. Take care. Never ever give up.

Kusal Goonewardena

IS YOUR LIFE ON HOLD?

Our enthusiasm for life can come to a painful halt when physical limitations put an offending barrier to the human spirit, not allowing us to experience new thrills and adventure. Every individual wishes to experience greater joys and pleasures in life, getting that envied sense of thrill and emancipation through adventure. And there is nothing more frustrating than when our own body thwarts that ambition.

Low back pain has engulfed millions in its vicious wrap and continues to do so with each advancing day. Read on if you too have that urge to go out and live your life to the hilt, but feel handicapped with low back pain playing a spoilsport!

Keep a keen eye on the signs your body is giving you and forge ahead with this book to seek help. It's not the end of the world and we have methods that can lead you on your way to safe recovery and healing. You can once again relish the true joys of living, without any physical limitations putting a dampener on your cherished zest for a good life.

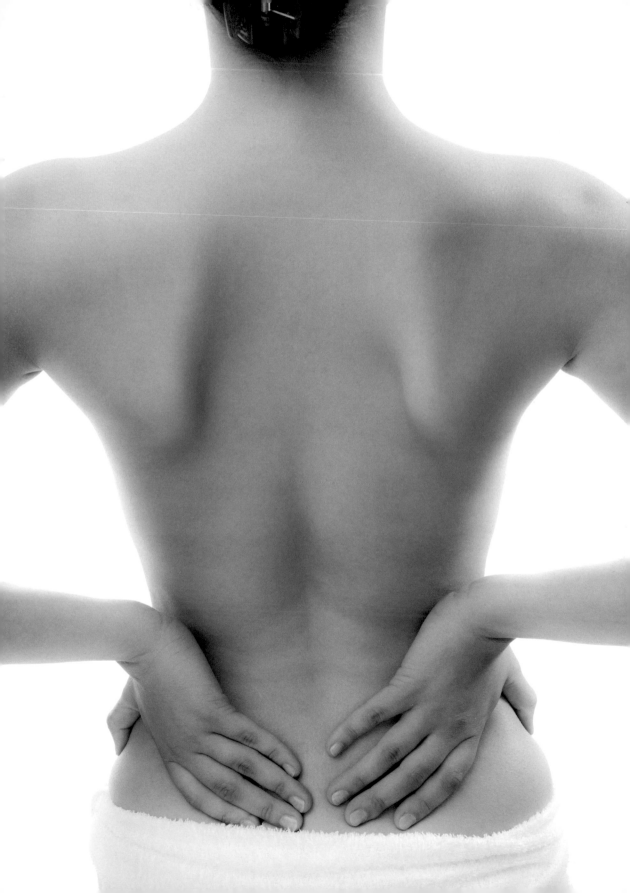

CONTENTS

CONTENTS

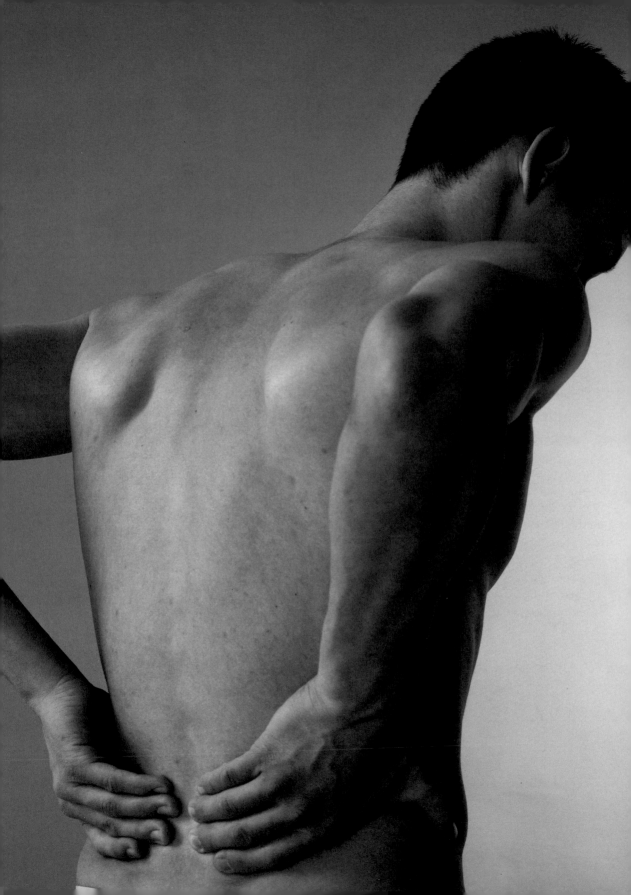

INTRODUCTION

By its typical definition, low back pain (LBP) can be a sudden, sharp, persistent or dull pain that is felt below the waist. Your back is one of the most sensitive, yet heavily used parts of the body. It literally carries the whole burden of your existence. It is with the early signs of pain in the lumbar region or the lower back that you begin to see the first signs of the wear and tear that this complicated structure has been going through.

In fact, low back pain is one of the very few forms of pain that can hugely vary in its intensity. The pain in your low back can often range from a mild, dull and annoying pain, to a disabling pain that is persistent and very intense. The latter category of pain can be severely debilitating and can strongly interfere with an individual's normal functioning.

THE TIME FACTOR

The most conspicuous and significant fact of low back pain is that it might not develop suddenly in a short span of time due to any one prominent reason. Instead, the condition might develop over a long course of time, after you've been performing many physical activities in the wrong manner, such as sitting, standing, sleeping, lifting and the like. Once developed, there is then an immediate onset of the pain once a triggering incident takes place, such as a sudden fall, jerk or an accident.

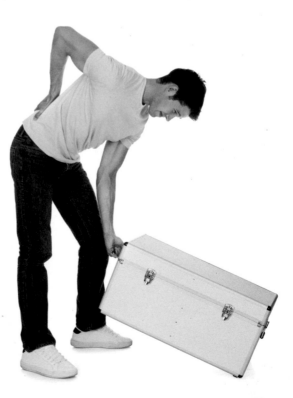

LOW BACK – THE STRUCTURE

The human spine is one of the most complex structures, comprised of a series of components that each have its own essential function. In fact, it is the spine that performs the all-important function of giving shape and structure to the body, apart from providing all the required support. It is primarily for this reason that an episode of low back pain can hinder your efficiency in daily life as nothing else can.

When attempting to understand what exactly is happening to your body as you suffer from LBP and why it is happening to you, it is first important that you understand the basic structure of the spine.

The human spine is made up of small bones, known as vertebrae that are heaped up on top of each other. The following is a brief introduction of various parts of the human spine.

The human spine is one of the most complex structures, comprised of a series of components that each have its own essential function

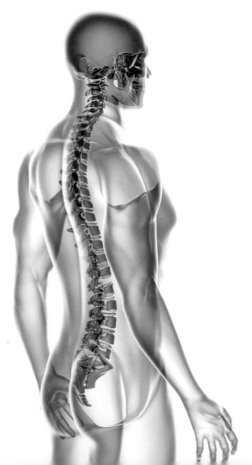

Vertebrae

The vertebrae are small bones that connect together to create a canal that protects the spinal cord. The spinal column basically comprises three sections which create natural curves in the back, including the:

- Neck area (Cervical)
- Chest area (Thoracic)
- Lower back (Lumbar)

Meanwhile, the lower section of your spine is comprised of vertebrae that are fused together. In addition, five lumbar vertebrae connect the upper spine to the pelvis.

Spinal Cord and Nerves

These are basically the electrical cables that travel through the spinal canal and carry messages between the brain and muscles. It is through openings of the vertebrae that the nerves stem out from the spinal cord.

Muscles and Ligaments

The muscles and ligaments offer support and stability to your spine, along with the upper body. Strong ligaments perform the important function of connecting your vertebrae and helping to keep the spinal column in its accurate position.

Facet Joints

In between the vertebrae, small joints are located that help the spine to move. These facet joints are located extremely close to the spinal nerves.

Intervertebral discs

These are the small components of the human spine that sit in between the vertebrae. When you run or walk, these intervertebral discs act as shock absorbers and prevent the vertebrae from rubbing against each other. Along with the facet joints, they perform the function of helping the spine to move, twist and bend.

The intervertebral discs are basically made of two basic components:

- **Annulus fibrosus, which is the tough and flexible outer ring of the disc**
- **Nucleus pulposus, which is the soft, jelly-like center of the annulus fibrosus, giving the disc its shock-absorbing capabilities**

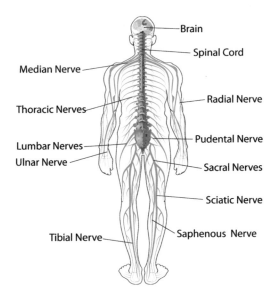

Brain
Spinal Cord
Median Nerve
Radial Nerve
Thoracic Nerves
Pudental Nerve
Lumbar Nerves
Ulnar Nerve
Sacral Nerves
Sciatic Nerve
Saphenous Nerve
Tibial Nerve

BACK PAIN – THE EPIDEMIC

If you too have suffered from the agonising impacts of low back pain, then you can take solace from the fact that LBP impacts a major segment of the world population. The National Institutes of Health (NIH) reports that at least 75% to 85% of people will suffer from low back pain at least once in their lifetime. The reports also state back pain is the most frequent cause behind the hindering of normal activity levels in adults younger than 45 years of age.

Increased instances of undesirable lifestyles and overall drooping standards of health have led to low back pain assuming almost epidemic proportions in the last few years. In fact, a whopping 66% of adult Americans are said to be suffering from recurring back pain, with numbers surely on an upward trend.

Research also indicates that 8 out of every 10 Canadians suffer from low back pain at some point in their life. It is the second leading cause of time loss at work in Canada. Back pain actually amounts to the costliest cause of time loss from work in the region.

Another study reports LBP to be the cause of expenditure amounting to a staggering $16 billion, out of the total of $27 billion incurred on musculoskeletal problems.

YOUR ACTION PLAN

Correct and timely decisions taken now can save you a lot of suffering later and might even help in a speedy recovery from an episode of LBP. An action plan for an LBP patient should be similar to the following presentation.

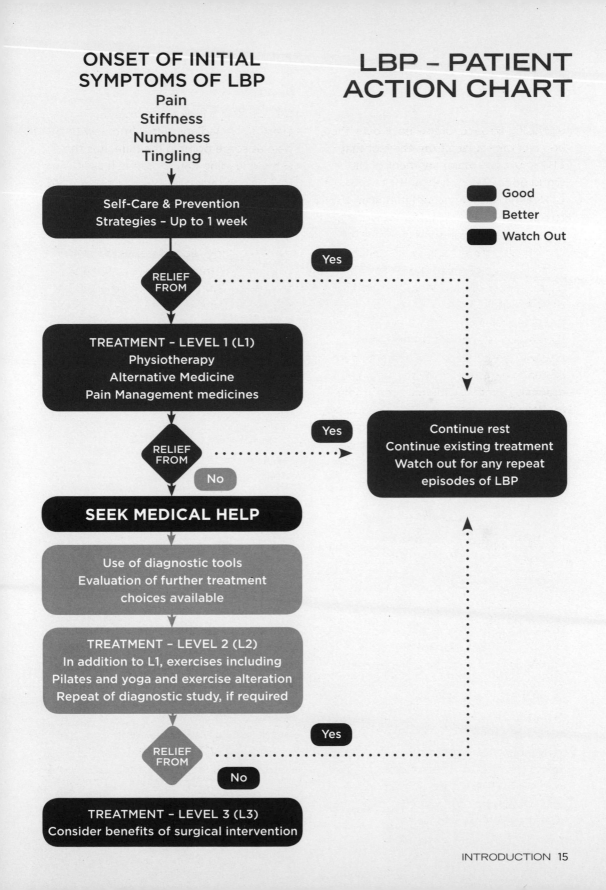

ONSET OF INITIAL SYMPTOMS OF LBP
Pain
Stiffness
Numbness
Tingling

LBP – PATIENT ACTION CHART

Good
Better
Watch Out

Self-Care & Prevention Strategies – Up to 1 week

RELIEF FROM — **Yes**

TREATMENT – LEVEL 1 (L1)
Physiotherapy
Alternative Medicine
Pain Management medicines

RELIEF FROM — **Yes**

No

SEEK MEDICAL HELP

Use of diagnostic tools
Evaluation of further treatment choices available

TREATMENT – LEVEL 2 (L2)
In addition to L1, exercises including Pilates and yoga and exercise alteration
Repeat of diagnostic study, if required

RELIEF FROM — **Yes**

No

TREATMENT – LEVEL 3 (L3)
Consider benefits of surgical intervention

Continue rest
Continue existing treatment
Watch out for any repeat episodes of LBP

In order to achieve the results from the patient action chart on page 15, there needs to be effective communication between the patient and the physician. The openness and clarity of communication between the two needs to be established and maintained as a foundation for a successful treatment plan for low back pain.

PATIENT – THERAPIST RELATIONSHIP

PATIENT CHART		THERAPIST CHART	
Inputs to Doctor	Primary Responsibility	Inputs to Patient	Primary Responsibility
1 Detail of symptoms, basis, Back Pain Journal page 111 2 Detail of medical history	1 Compliance of physician's instructions 2 Convey honest feedback about treatment 3 Regular visits to convey feedback 4 Regular self-care	1 To give full knowledge of the working of spine/lower back 2 Explanation of exact cause 3 To give complete knowledge of the treatment plan	1 To accept details of feedback and alter treatment plan, if required 2 To give the patient a true picture of the state of health

SELF-ANALYSIS

Low back pain can become a very intimidating condition for someone not too familiar with the anatomy of the human body and the lower back in general. In such conditions, it is important to make a note of your most prominent signs and symptoms. Once you have the record of these symptoms, you can then report them to your healthcare provider who will then diagnose the type of pain you have along with the corrective measures you need to take.

You can use the Back Pain Journal on page 111 to record the patterns and vital symptoms of your health. Take it to your physician who can then understand and analyse your condition well.

In addition, you can also use this journal to carry out a self-analysis of your condition and improvements.

Once you have the record of
these symptoms, you can then
report them to your healthcare
provider who will then diagnose
the type of pain you have along
with the corrective measures
you need to take.

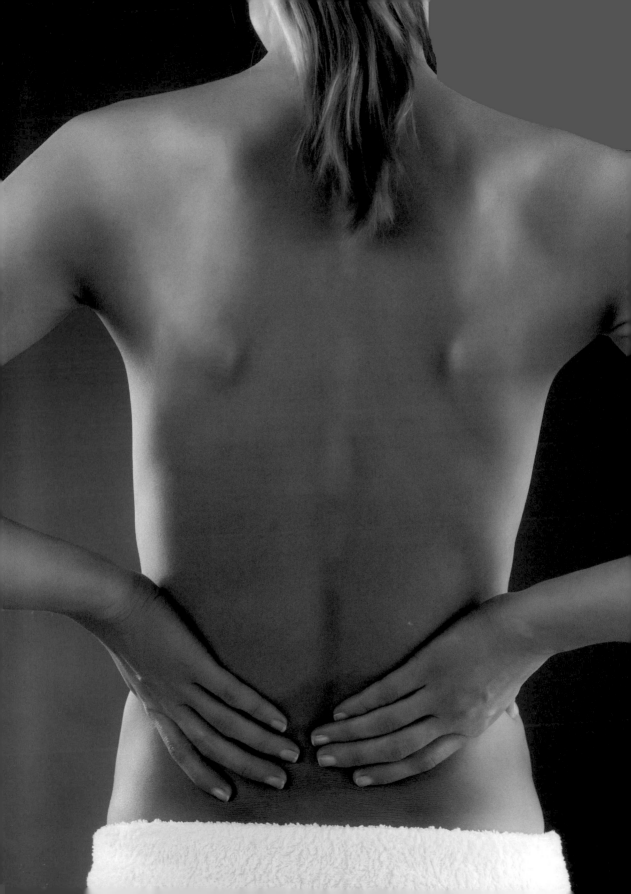

LOW BACK PAIN - TYPES, SIGNS AND SYMPTOMS

TYPES OF LOW BACK PAIN

Low back pain is one of the most widespread forms of pain–related disorders. This further leads to a vast range of variation in the form of pain that occurs, which can be understood on the basis of different parameters.

In the following section I've given a brief outline of the various types of low back pain basis: the duration, cause, and location of the pain.

BASIS OF DURATION

The duration of pain is the most commonly used method to differentiate between different types of low back pain. In fact, the duration of the pain, along with its severity helps the physician to decide on the exact cause of the pain and the treatment modalities required.

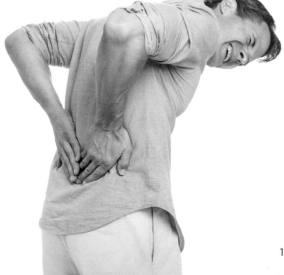

The following is a description of each of the three types of low back pain based on their duration.

Acute Pain

Acute back pain is basically a short term pain, mostly lasting from a few days to a few weeks (basically four weeks to the maximum). Symptoms associated with acute back pain can sometimes become serious if left untreated.

Sub Acute Pain

Sub acute back pain is a moderate level of pain that lasts from anywhere between 4 and 12 weeks and presents itself in occasional flare-ups of pain.

Chronic Pain

Chronic back pain is a pain that typically lasts for more than three months. This form of pain might be progressive in nature i.e. it might develop gradually over time. Alternatively, this form of pain might suddenly increase to a higher level after short gaps and then the level of pain might return to normal.

BASIS OF TREATMENT MODALITIES

On the basis of the treatment that is generally required, experts suggest two different types of low back pain, including mechanical pain and inflammatory pain, both being sub-divisions of non-specific pain, also known as NS-LBP.

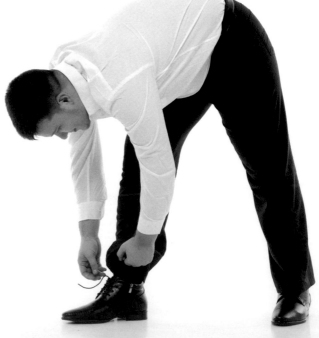

WHY THE PAIN IN MY BACK?
THE LATEST CLINICAL FINDINGS

The latest research in pain shows that it is more of a signal by the brain that something is not working properly in the body. In short, pain in the body works very much like the red engine dashboard light in a car. When the engine is not functioning properly then the light on the dashboard lights up. When it lights up we naturally assume something is wrong with the car, therefore we take it to the mechanic, they help fix the engine and that stops the red dashboard light. When you suffer from back pain it is the same thing — the red dashboard light is in the back. To fix the light, we have to fix the engine. The engine is the whole body. In the past many sufferers from back pain have thought that their problem is in the lower back, and most of the treatment has occurred here. However in as many as 75% of cases the problem occurs elsewhere, other than the back. In only 25% of cases does the problem actually occur in the lower back, therefore causing pain here.

Signs and Symptoms

The severity of symptoms of low back pain are directly dependent on how long the underlying problem was ignored for. For example, if the cause of the back pain was a tight joint in the upper spine, and this was ignored over time by getting intermittent, short term treatment, then the signs and symptoms can be much worse. There are three phases to the signs and symptoms a person may feel. First they may notice tightness or stiffness in the lower back, (people tend to ignore this) and then the body continues to warn the person by then making movements apprehensive. For example, a person who wants to bend forward and tie their shoelaces will feel uncomfortable to move down quickly into the position they want. This is apprehension and is usually ignored as a symptom. Finally it is pain. This is when people usually think that something is actually wrong. By this time they are further down the injury path, but the good news is it might not be too late to find a solution for them.

Pain that worsens while coughing, twisting, sneezing or after sitting for a prolonged duration

Did you know?

It has often been observed that the severity of the symptoms of LBP might not correlate directly with the severity of the problem. This implies that strong symptoms might not essentially indicate that any strong underlying disorder exists. For instance, a simple muscle strain might cause extreme pain; while on the other hand, a disc that is completely degenerated might not cause any pain at all.

There are a number of symptoms of LBP which are quite generic in nature and are seen in almost all of the cases. The most prominent amongst these include:

- Severe pain
- Stiffness
- Tingling
- Numbness

Pain, that

- Radiates towards buttocks or legs
- Worsens while coughing, twisting, sneezing or after sitting for a prolonged duration

SPECIFIC SYMPTOMS

The symptoms and signs of LBP usually emanate from three basic causes, indicating the exact location of the problem. The following are the exact symptoms of LBP in specific correlation with each of these conditions.

Signs associated with muscle strains and joint stiffness

Being the most common cause of LBP, injuries and sprains in the muscles present the most prominent symptoms. Such an injury or sprain of the muscle usually presents in the form of the following symptoms:

- Cramping or muscle spasms
- Stiffness, at times inability to move
- Pain in buttocks
- Pain that aggravates with certain movements but feels better with rest
- Very tight muscles on either side of the lower spine

If your LBP has emanated from a muscle strain, then the pain will normally last from one to three days. This period will then be followed by a few days or weeks of moderate pain as the inflammation diminishes and the affected portion begins to heal.

Signs associated with nerve root pressure

If your low back pain has been caused due to nerve root pressure, then the most prominent symptom is that the pain travels down the sciatic nerve in the back of the leg, also known as sciatica or radiculopathy. The most conspicuous signs of the pain caused by nerve root compression include:

- Pain that is accompanied by numbness, tingling, weakness or loss of specific reflexes
- Pain that is present only on one side
- Pain that aggravates due to long periods of sitting or standing
- Pain that is quite sharp and is accompanied by a burning sensation

The most critical warning signs, also known as the 'red flags' include: severe fever, nausea, vomiting, abdominal pain, weakness or sweating

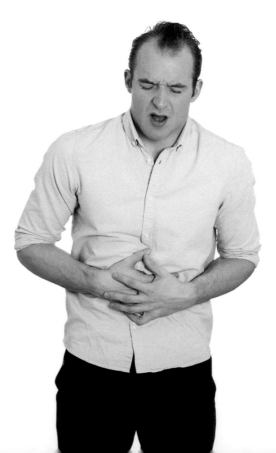

THE RED FLAGS

Though low back pain can rarely be a cause for panic or alarm, there are a number of red flags or warning signs that need immediate medical attention in case they surface. The most critical warning signs, also known as the 'red flags' include:

- Back pain that is accompanied with loss of bladder or bowel control
- Loss of sensation in the legs or arms
- Numbness around the genitals, buttocks or anus
- Pain that aggravates when you cough or bend forward from the waist
- Pain that radiates down the leg, towards the knee
- Presence of high fever, which is an indicator of a spinal infection
- Pain that travels up towards the chest
- Severe pain with weight loss, caused by a tumor in the spine
- Severe fever, nausea, vomiting, abdominal pain, weakness or sweating
- Treatment shows no or negligible effect after 2-3 weeks

In addition, individuals who meet the following conditions and suffer from frequent episodes of low back pain also need to seek medical help immediately. This criterion includes individuals who:

- Are either under 20 or over 55 years of age
- Have suffered from a recent accident, injury or trauma
- Have consumed steroids for a few months
- Are a drug abuser
- Have been suffering from cancer
- Have a low immune system due to treatments like chemotherapy or diseases like HIV/AIDS and the like

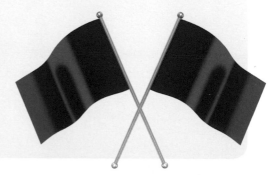

RISK FACTORS

Research shows that a majority of adults experience low back pain at some point in their lives. However, a certain section of individuals are more prone to getting episodes of low back pain. Here are the main risk factors which make an individual more vulnerable to developing LBP.

- **Employees in construction jobs or other places involving heavy lifting**
- **Employees in jobs involving lots of bending, twisting or vibration of the whole body, such as those using a sandblaster**
- **Individuals maintaining poor postural habits over a long period of time**
- **Pregnant women**
- **Individuals above the age of 30, especially having an unhealthy lifestyle**
- **Individuals who do not exercise regularly or are overweight**
- **Individuals who smoke regularly**
- **Patients of arthritis, osteoporosis**
- **Patients of anxiety or depression**
- **Individuals with a low pain tolerance level**

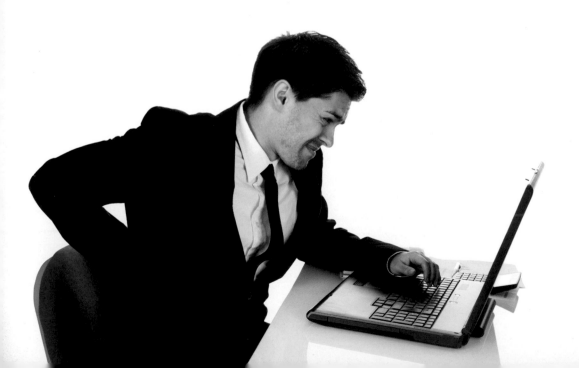

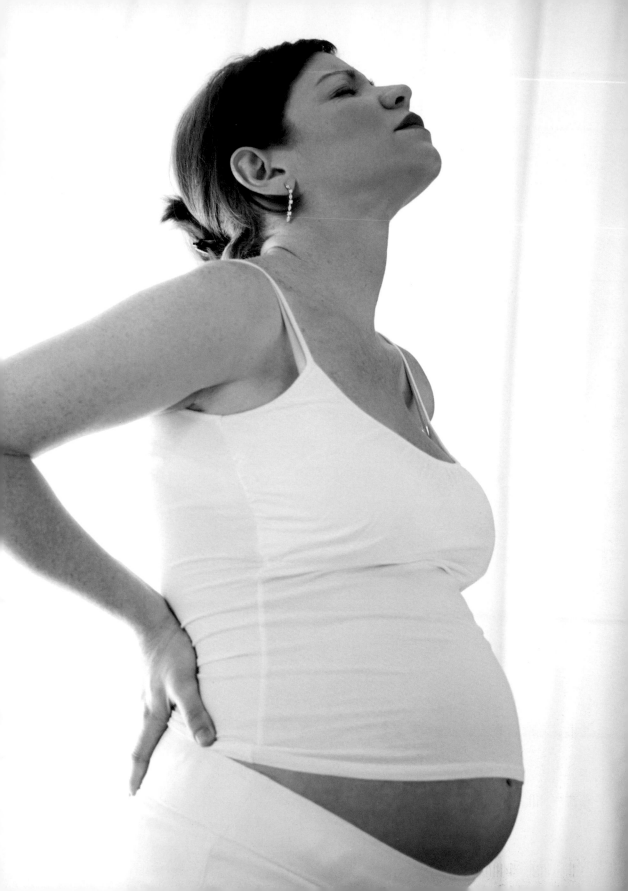

CASE STUDY 1

Jessica, 34 years old

Mother of two children and the youngest being only six months started suffering from acute low back pain every morning and at night.

She could not get to sleep, had difficulties finding a good resting position and the pain was aggravated by breastfeeding and when the baby was crying.

Treatment – Her pain was mainly due to poor posture in her upper back. The poor posture was exacerbated during the breastfeeding as she always bent down and forwards for the baby, instead of bringing the baby to her breast. Helping her be aware of this improved her condition remarkably. She started feeding in a seat that had arm rests and she had proper back support throughout her spine – from her lower back right to the level of her shoulders. She combined this with regular yoga for relaxation (two 30 minute sessions per week from home) and her pain was under control in five days.

The poor posture was exacerbated during the breastfeeding as she always bent down and forwards for the baby, instead of bringing the baby to her breast

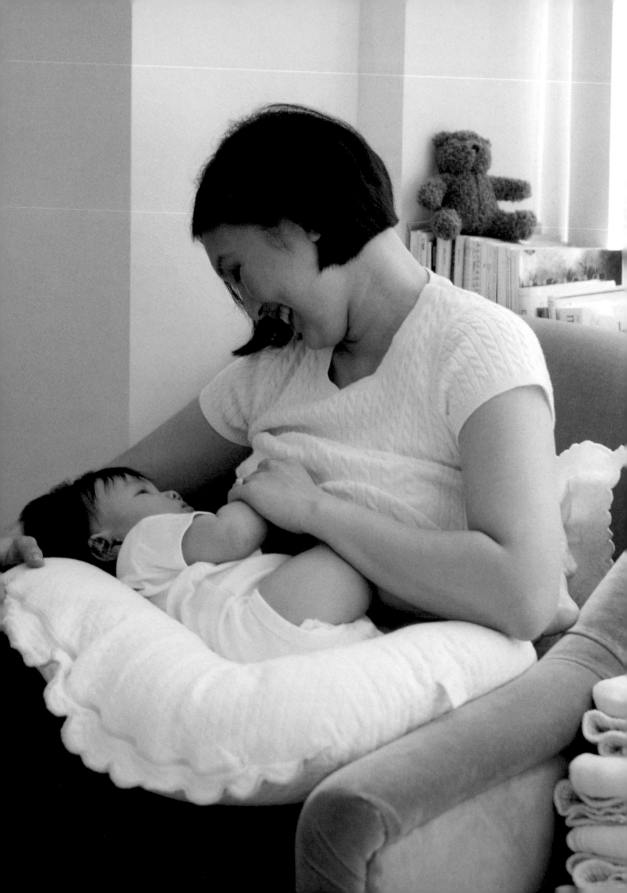

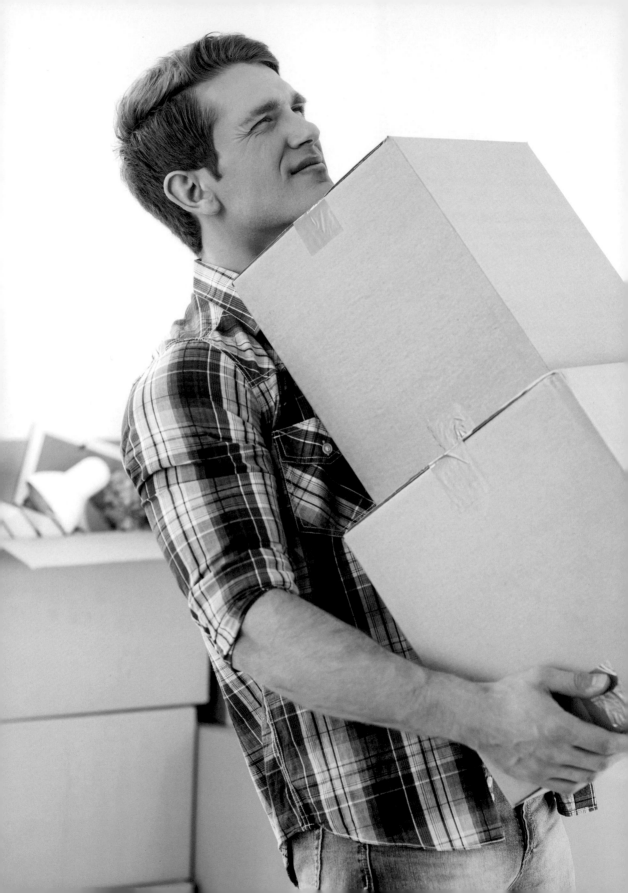

LOW BACK PAIN – KEY CAUSES

Have you ever suffered strong bouts of low back pain but have felt helpless when it comes to understanding the exact cause? In many cases low back pain is not a disorder in itself but often a symptom of another disease or malfunction you might be suffering from.

To understand how low back pain finds its roots in your body, it is first important to understand how your body and bones react to the ageing process. As your age progresses, there is a significant drop in the levels of bone strength and muscle elasticity. Soon after, the discs start to lose their flexibility and the fluid levels begin to diminish. Eventually, this decreases the ability of your discs to cushion the vertebrae appropriately.

Beyond a series of elaborate analysis and research findings, a sudden, improper use of the postural muscles emerges as the single most common reason of low back pain. When you do not engage the proper posture when performing tasks that require extra effort the result is sudden onset of pain in the back. Such activities could span across a vast range

from playing an unplanned game of tennis, doing the gardening, lifting heavy furniture, having a fall to being in a car accident.

For better understanding, I'll discuss various activities, medical conditions and disorders that might cause LBP under several sub-categories.

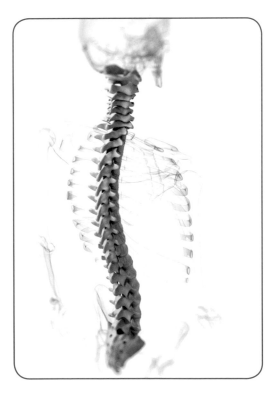

INJURIES AND ACTIVITIES

Your back bears the direct impact of your physical activity and will present an immediate impact in case of any injury or accident. In fact, research reports that at least 75% of cases of low back pain occur due to the lumbar strain or musculo-ligamentous sprains. In the course of everyday life, there are five important and common causes which mark the onset of low back pain for most of the individuals. These include:

1 **Improper conditioning of the postural muscles**

2 **Improper lifting techniques**

3 **Sprains and injuries of the ligaments and muscles, such as lumbosacral strain, intervertebral joint injuries and rupture of intervertebral discs**

4 **Sudden impact such as from a car accident**

NERVE ROOT COMPRESSION

Various medical conditions or disorders in the human body can lead to an additional pressure being put on the nerve roots in the spinal canal. This can further lead to a mild to strong episode of low back pain, lasting for varying durations.

Your low back pain could be a result of nerve root compression if you are diagnosed with any of the following medical conditions:

Herniated/Bulging Disc

Individuals involved in repetitive activities having a lot of vibration or motion are prone to developing a herniated disc. If you've been extensively engaged in machine use or a specific sports activity requiring heavy physical exertion or have attempted to lift a heavy object using inappropriate lifting techniques, then you could actually be suffering from a herniated disc, which in turn might be an underlying cause of your low back pain.

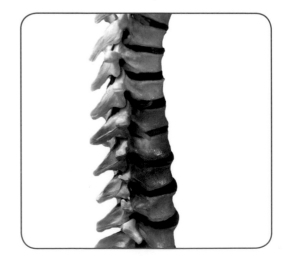

Osteoarthritis

Also known as joint degeneration, osteoarthritis is mostly related to age and affects the small facet joints in the spine, ultimately leading to episodes of low back pain. Interestingly, research shows that osteoarthritis affects nearly thrice the number of women than it affects men.

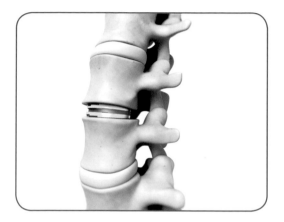

Spondylolysis

This category of physical disorder is basically a vertebra defect that can allow a vertebra to slide over another one and lead to pain in the back. This particular condition gets aggravated due to certain specific physical activities that might put stress on the affected regions.

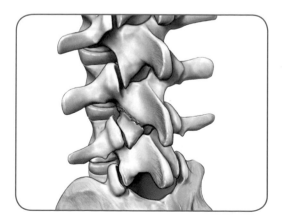

Lumbar Spinal Stenosis

This category of physical disorder is a medical condition which occurs when the space around the spinal cord gets narrowed. This further puts pressure on the spinal cord as well as the spinal nerve roots, eventually leading to pain, numbness or weakness in the legs.

When the spinal stenosis occurs in the lower back, it is called lumbar spinal stenosis, which usually results from the normal aging process. With age, the soft tissues and bones in the spine harden on their own or even become overgrown. Such degenerative changes may narrow the space around the spinal cord and eventually cause spinal stenosis.

In addition, other conditions such as fractures of the vertebrae and spinal deformities such as curvature problems could also cause compression on the nerve roots, further leading to low back pain.

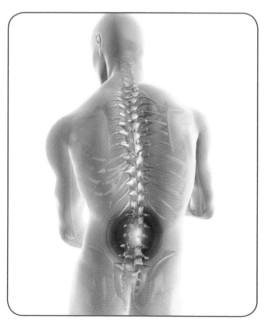

SPINAL CONDITIONS

In addition to the previous causes, there are other medical conditions, specifically related to the spine, that can lead to low back pain in some individuals, though the incidence is not very high. Read on for a brief description of each of these conditions:

- **Spinal tumors, which are basically growths that develop on the bones and ligaments of the spine or the nerve roots**
- **Metastatic tumors from other points such as prostate, lungs, kidney and intestine**
- **Ankylosing spondylitis, which is a kind of arthritis that mostly affects the spine**
- **Bacterial infections, such as osteomyelitis, which is an infection of the bone or other infections in the spinal discs or spinal cord occurring due to IV drug use, surgeries or other injection treatments**
- **Paget's disease, leading to abnormal bone growth, which further affects the pelvis, spine, skull, cheat and lungs**
- **Scheuermann's disease, basically a disorder in which one or more of the vertebrae begin to develop wedge-shaped deformities, further leading to conditions like curvature in the spine, eventually leading to low back pain**

FUNCTIONAL PROBLEMS

Low back pain can often occur due to a number of functional issues associated with activities of everyday life. Here are some of the most common functional problems causing low back pain:

- **Pregnancy, childbirth and gynecological operations**
- **Uterus prolapse**
- **Pelvic inflammatory diseases**
- **Cancerous lesions in the pelvic regions**
- **Endometriosis**
- **Obesity**
- **Short leg (on one side)**

OTHER CONDITIONS

Some of the other conditions that might cause low back pain include:

- **Peptic ulcers**
- **Aortic aneurysm**
- **Gallbladder disease**
- **Pancreatitis**
- **Cauda equine syndrome**
- **Urinary disorders**
- **Kidney disorders**
- **Biliary stones**
- **Prostate disease**

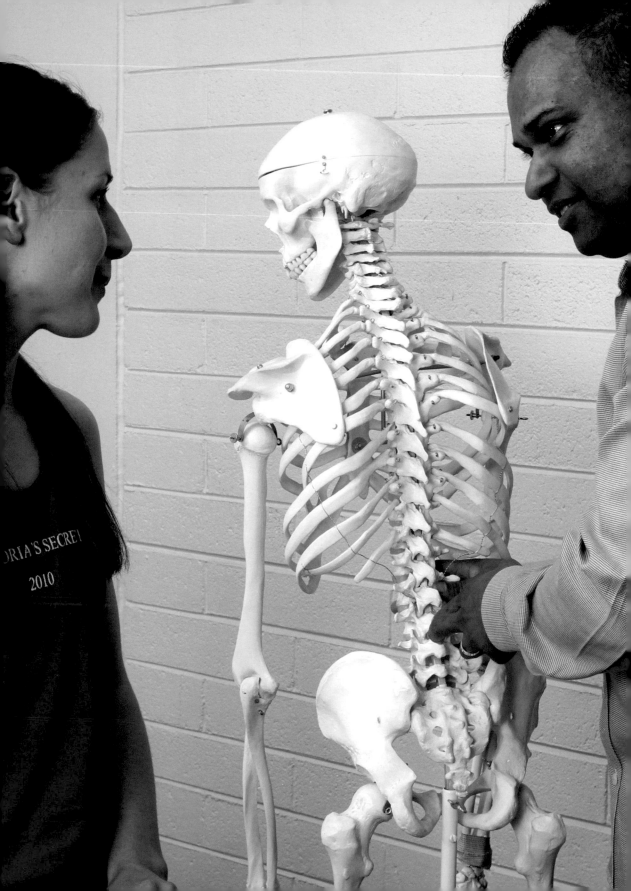

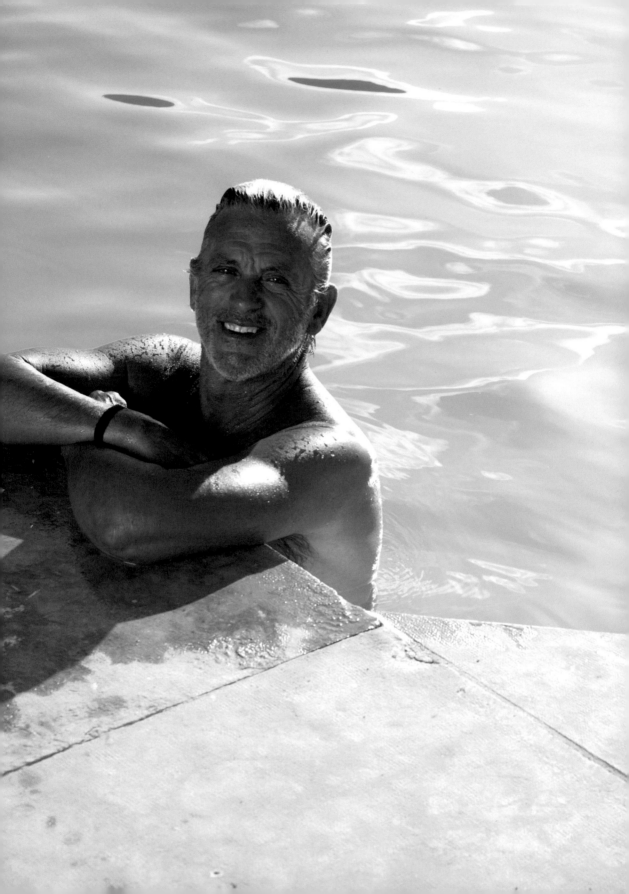

CASE STUDY 2

Adam, 48 years old

Adam was a mechanic who suffered from pain during work and when at home. He was a strong gentleman who had been a mechanic for more than 25 years. His pain was gradual and now it was so bad that he couldn't even sit for more than 20 minutes.

Treatment – Due to his consistent hard work he did not have time for exercise or sport. He was always moving in a forward bending manner (for his work) and this meant that crucial muscles and joints that help move the spine sideways were not being utilised. A treatment program to address these joints in his lumbar spine and a stretching program from his gluteal muscel group improved his condition by 60%. Further to this a regular swimming program (only one 30 minute session every week) allowed him to improve his condition to over 85%. He needs regular tune ups with his therapist — every month when he is busy at work, otherwise every 3 months when he has his back pain under control.

A treatment program to address these joints in his lumbar spine and a stretching program from his gluteal muscel group improved his condition by 60%. Further to this a regular swimming program (only one 30 minute session every week) allowed him to improve his condition to over 85%

CAUSES OF LBP

Injuries and Activities

1. Improper conditioning of postural muscles

2. Improper lifting techniques

3. Sprains and injuries of ligaments and muscles

4. Sudden impact

Nerve Root Compression

1. Herniated disc

2. Osteoarthritis

3. Spondylolysis

4. Lumbar Spinal Stenosis

5. Sciatica

Spinal Conditions

1. Spinal and metastatic tumors

2. Ankylosing Spondylities

3. Bacterial infections, e.g. Osteomyelitis

4. Paget's disease

5. Scheuermann's disease

Functional Problems

1. Pregnancy, childbirth, gynecological operations

2. Uterus prolapse

3. Pelvic inflammatory diseases

4. Cancerous lesions in pelvic regions

5. Endometriosis

6. Obesity

7. Short leg

Others

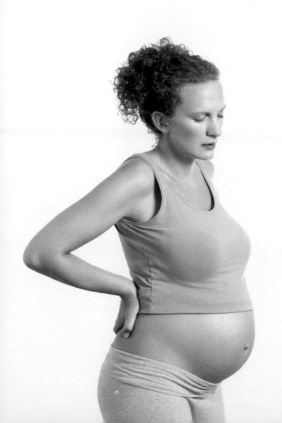

1. Peptic ulcers

2. Aortic aneurysm

3. Gallbladder disease

4. Pancreatitis

5. Cauda equine syndrome

6. Urinary disorders

7. Kidney disorders

8. Biliary stones

9. Prostate disease

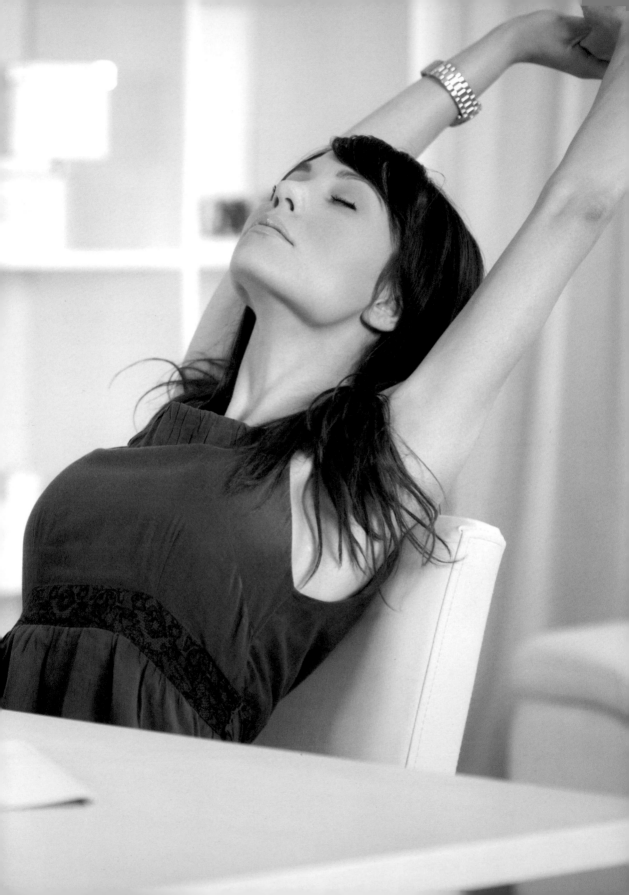

SELF-CARE AND PREVENTION

SELF-CARE

Medical research has always reinforced the need for better preventive measures as against rigorous treatment methods. Even in the course of your everyday life, there are a number of precautions and preventive measures you can follow to avoid causing a strain on your back.

Read on for some of the most important points to remember in order to avoid hurting your back, which can further lead to a strong bout of low back pain.

PREVENTIVE MEASURES

1 Remember not to bend while trying to lift something from the ground. Instead, try to bend your knees and squat to pick an object. Keeping the back straight, hold the object close to your body and then try to lift it up

2 While moving heavy objects, try to push instead of pull

3 Take frequent breaks to stretch if you need to sit at your desk or drive for longer durations of time

4 Follow a regular regimen for exercise as a sedentary and inactive lifestyle contributes to low back pain substantively

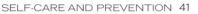

CURATIVE MEASURES

. . . .

1 **Remain as active as possible during the course of LBP. Prolonged periods of bed rest have been known to be a causative factor of low back pain**

2 **Follow a home exercise program soon after the initial pain has subsided**

3 **Use a heat pad or ice pack (whichever helps you the most) to relieve your pain, especially in the first few weeks**

4 **Lumbar supports such as back support, corsets and braces might also be helpful in alleviating pain**

5 **Try to sleep with a pillow placed between or under your knees**

6 **During an attack of acute back pain, try to practice deep breathing. Rhythmic and slow breathing calms the mind, allowing the body to enter into a more relaxed state**

7 **Try to perform light stretching exercises several times a day**

Experts strongly warn about creating an undue stressful environment in context to your low back pain. Worrying in excess over how bad your pain is, when it is going to heal and how much it is going to affect your efficiency will actually harm you all the more instead of offering any healing benefits.

POSTURE MANAGEMENT

As you rush around the day performing the basic duties of your working hours, there are a number of postures you take, which if faulty can lead to low back pain.

The most common postures that need attention include:

Sitting

Standing

Sleeping

Walking

Read on for a brief set of guidelines that demonstrate what are the right postures that should be used to sit, stand and sleep in order to avoid getting low back pain.

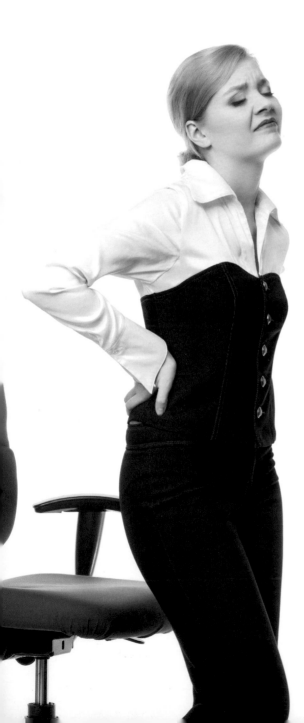

SITTING

Following are the most important guidelines for sitting in the right posture:

■ **Whenever possible, sit only in chairs with straight backs, or those that offer a support to the lower back**

■ **Always try to keep your knees at a bit higher platform than your hips**

■ **When sitting at an odd level, use a low stool to keep your feet on**

■ **When you have to move while sitting, turn by moving your whole body, instead of twisting your waist**

■ **Sit straight and move your seat forward while driving. Keep a small pillow behind the lower back when driving for longer durations**

Always try to keep your knees at a bit higher platform than your hips

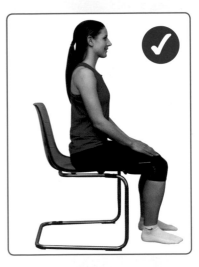

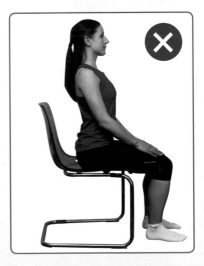

STANDING

Follow these simple guidelines for correct standing posture in order to avoid damage to your lower back:

- **Rest one foot on a low stool when standing for longer durations and switch the resting foot every 5 to 10 minutes**

- **Follow the standard dictum of a good standing posture, with your ears, shoulders and hips in a straight line, besides keeping your head up**

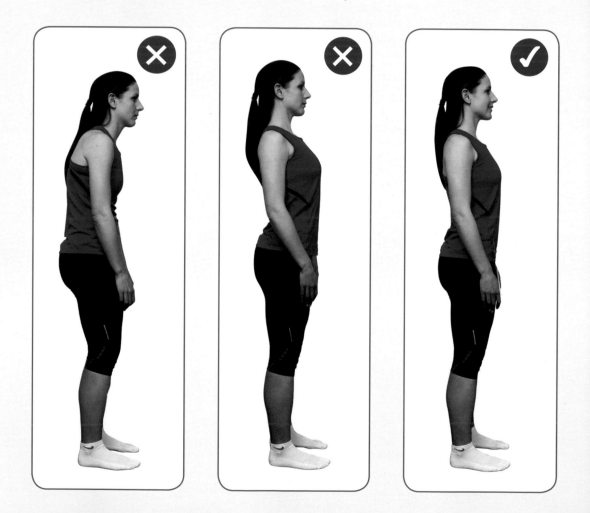

SLEEPING

While sleeping on your side with knees bent is the best posture, there are additional guidelines that can be of immense help, which include the following:

- **Use a pillow to support your neck**

- **Keep a pillow under your knees and another small one under the lower back, especially if you sleep on your back**

- **Always use a mattress which is less than 8 years old, unless they have a longer warranty period**

Keep a pillow under your knees and another small one under the lower back, especially if you sleep on your back

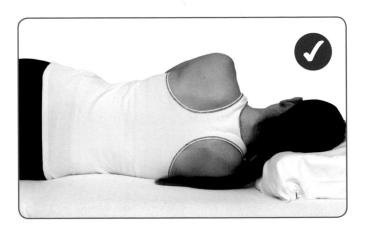

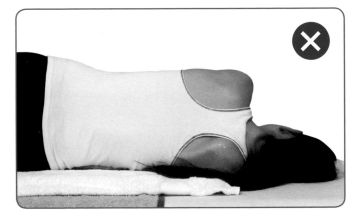

WALKING

When walking it is important to do the following

- **Look at the horizon**

- **Keep your chest bone up**

- **Elongate your spine and think 'tall' when you take steps**
- **Project your weight upwards and forwards instead of downwards**

Your posture will be tested when you are carrying a bag or heavy goods. Always try and check your posture in reflections e.g. at the bus stop, in shop front and building windows. Maintain your poise and balance, and this will help your posture.

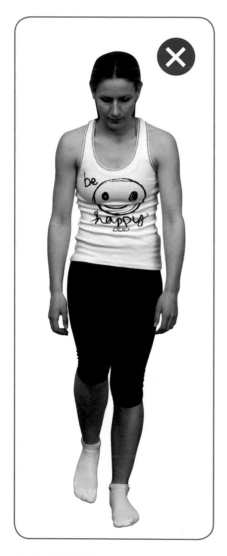 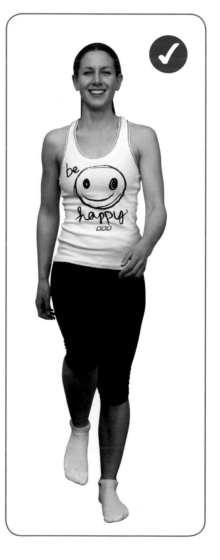

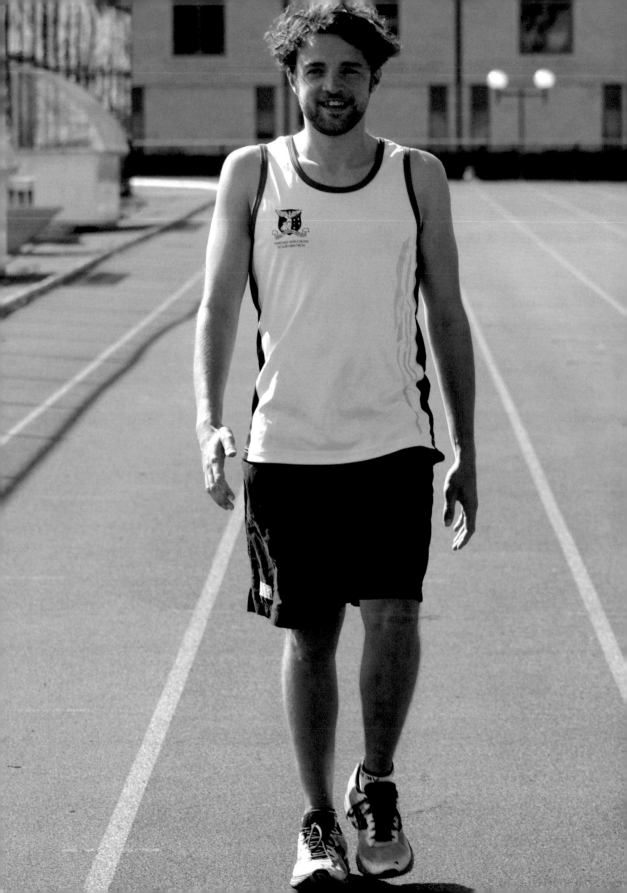

Try to incorporate as many antioxidant rich foods in your diet as possible. Foods such as green leafy vegetables and fruits such as blueberries, cherries and pomegranates are a good source of antioxidants.

NUTRITIONAL GUIDELINES

What diet you maintain and how you consume it actually determines the way your body shapes out. Low back pain is no exception to this rule and responds quite well to a planned and balanced dietary system.

Here I've listed some of the most important guidelines you need to observe daily in order to prevent as well as cure low back pain.

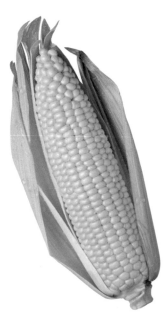

PRECAUTIONS

1 **LBP can often be triggered due to food sensitivities. Cut out any possible food allergens which may be in your diet. These include dairy, wheat or gluten, chocolate, corn, soy, preservatives or food additives such as alfalfa sprouts and onions**

2 **Try to incorporate as many antioxidant rich foods in your diet as possible. Foods such as green leafy vegetables and fruits such as blueberries, cherries and pomegranates are a good source of antioxidants**

3 **Refined foods such as white breads, pastas and sugar should be avoided as much as possible**

4 **Lean meats such as cold-water fish or products like beans should be consumed for more proteins instead of red meats**

5 **Healthy cooking oils such as olive oil or vegetable oil need to be used more**

6 **Reduce the intake of trans-fatty acids to the maximum possible extent. Common sources include bakery products such as cookies, crackers, cakes, onion rings, donuts and the like**

7 **Avoid intake of alcohol, tobacco and other such stimulants. Have at least 6-8 glasses of filtered water daily**

8 **Exercise for at least 30 minutes a day, minimum five days a week**

MEDICINAL SUPPLEMENTS

Including healthy nutritional supplements in your diet can be an added advantage when you are prone to be affected by low back pain. Here I've listed some of the most commonly suggested supplements, along with the specific benefit they offer:

- **For decreasing inflammation**
  Omega-3 fatty acid

- **For connective tissue support**
  Glucosamine/chondrotin

- **For bone strength**
  Calcium/Vitamin D supplements

HERBAL SUPPLEMENTS

Mostly available in the form of pills, capsules and tablets, which are the standardised and dried extracts, or as tinctures and liquid extracts, herbal concoctions are a useful preventive and curative measure for your low back pain. Read on for a quick list of the most important and beneficial herbal supplements available, along with their specific benefits:

- **For antioxidant and immune support**
  Ginko (Ginko biloba) extract

- **For antioxidant and immune effects**
  Green tea (Camelia sinensis)

- **For relief from pain and inflammation**
  Bromelain (Ananus comosus)
  Turmeric (Curcuma longa)
  Cat's claw (Uncaria tomentosa)
  Devil's claw (Harpagophytum procumbens)

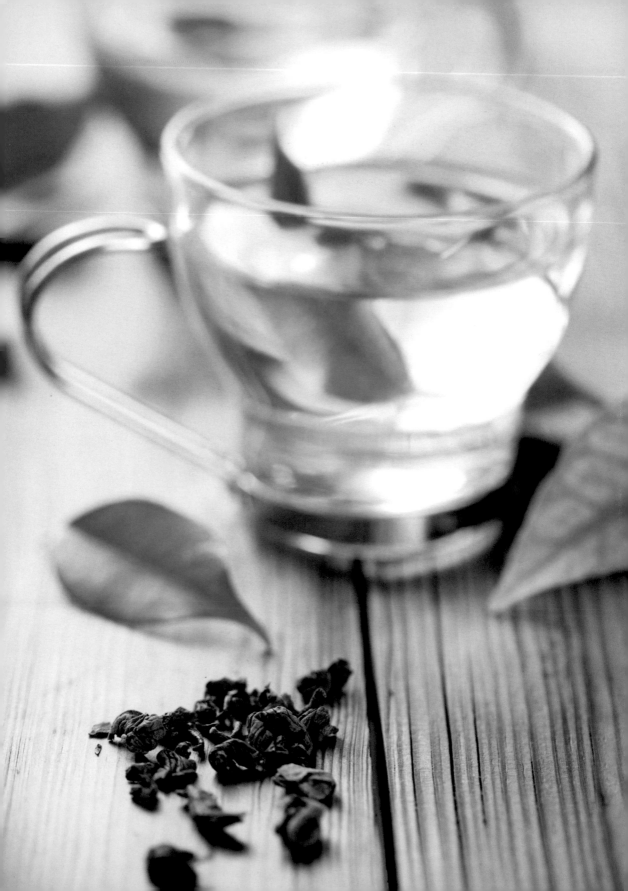

CASE STUDY 3

Jason, 44 years old

Jason was an accountant who suffered from low back pain every month and always during July. He couldn't sit for long periods, could not attend meetings that lasted more than 40 minutes and couldn't get comfortable in his seat.

He was an active person who went to the gym twice every week.

Treatment – Jason's problem was the nature of his work. His busiest periods were during the 'month end' where he had numerous deadlines for his accounting work. July was the end of the financial year where he would do 12-14 hour days. Once this was established an office exercise program was created to break up the heavy workload during the end of the month and during July. The exercise program involved keeping the spine mobile, keeping it moving and breaking up static postures. The whole routine would only last 2-3 minutes and would not affect his work. It was ascertained that if he could not manage his problem with the exercises that's when he would need to come in for treatment with his therapist. Proper ergonomics were also provided therefore his work desk and work chair were changed to be more user friendly. The computer screen was placed at the correct height and elbow rests on the chairs were provided to help maintain proper sitting posture.

The exercise program involved keeping the spine mobile, keeping it moving and breaking up static postures

CASE STUDY 4

Andrea, 67 years old

Andrea was a retiree who was very active on a daily basis around home. She spent 2-3 hours every day in the garden, maintaining the home and spending time on her hobby – knitting. Her back pain started during the spring months and by autumn it was quite unbearable.

Treatment – Andrea required five sessions with the physiotherapist and then to maintain her gains she started an exercise program that was called, 'stretches in the garden' and 'stretches before you knit'. This helped keep tight muscles and joints loose when she was in static postures e.g. kneeling at the flower bed or being seated for 1-2 hours knitting. She requires a tune up with her physiotherapist every season i.e. four times per year.

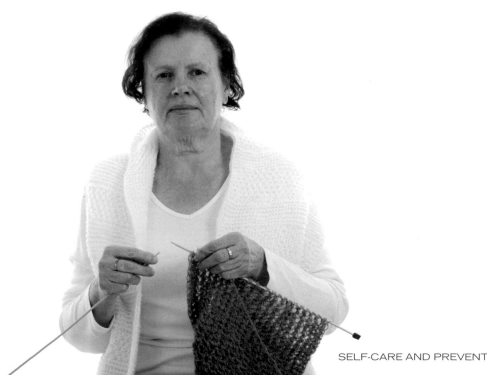

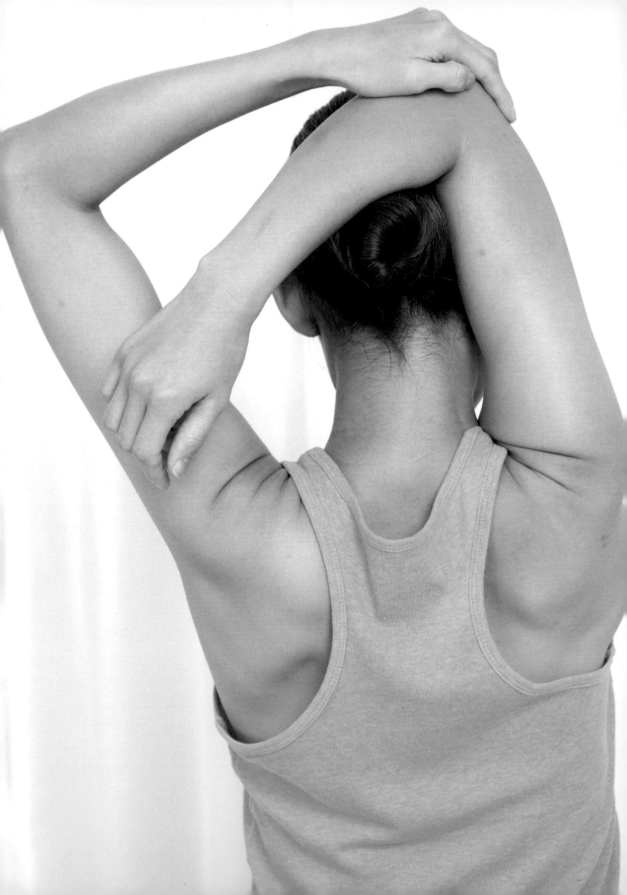

PHYSICAL THERAPY

PHYSIOTHERAPY EXERCISE PROGRAMS

An exercise program for reducing low back pain basically comprises of three main types of exercises, each having a different pre-set objective, including:

- **Postural Conditioning Exercises**

- **Stretching exercises**

- **Strengthening exercises**

- **Core exercises**

- **Aerobic exercises**

Before you begin your session of exercises of low back pain, make sure to do the following:

- **Do light aerobic exercises or take a brisk walk to warm up**

- **Place an exercise mat or a thick blanket on the floor where you plan to exercise**

- **Consult your physician, especially if you suffer from conditions like the herniated disc**

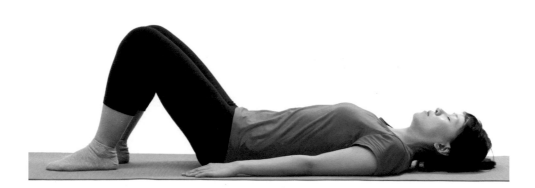

THE TOP 7 EXERCISES

PELVIC TILT

1

- Lie straight on your back

- Keep your feet flat and knees bent

- Push the small of your back into the floor by pulling the lower abdominal muscles up and inside

- Hold the back flat as you breathe in and out

- Hold for five seconds

- Repeat

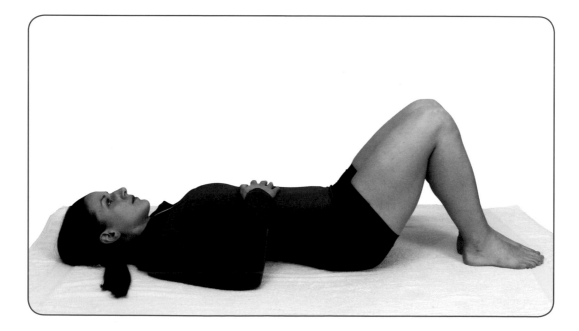

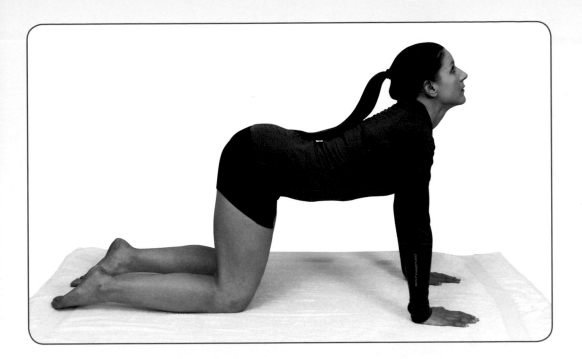

CAT AND CAMEL STRETCH

- Get down on all fours

- Position your hands under the shoulders and knees below your hips

- Let your head down

- Tuck your hips under and the middle of your back as high as you can

- Try to create a slight curve of your back towards the ceiling

- Hold the position for 5 seconds

- Once done, now try and sag your trunk as far as you can so that your back is arched, but do not pull it down

- Hold again for 5 seconds

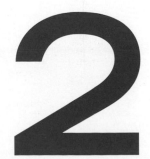

KNEE TO CHEST

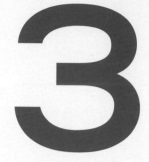

- Lie on your back on a table or any firm surface

- Hold your hands tightly behind the thigh

- Pull it towards your chest (pain permitting)

- Keep your opposite leg flat

- Hold for 30 seconds

- Switch legs and then repeat

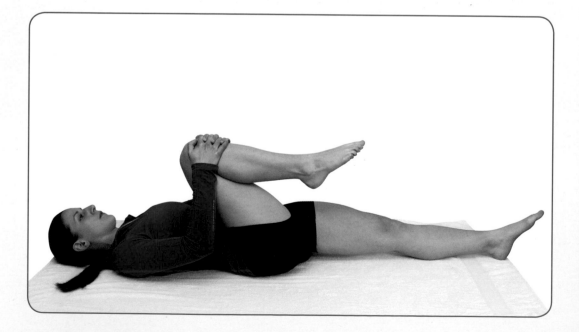

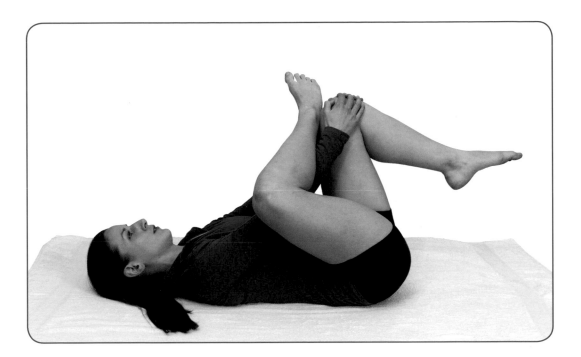

PIRIFORMIS STRETCH

- Lie down on the floor with one foot placed on the lateral aspect of the opposite side knee

- With your arm, gently try to pull the thigh of your bent leg and twist the body

- Hold for 30 seconds

- Repeat with same side for 3-5 times

- Repeat with other leg

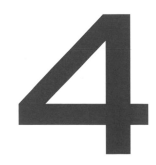

HAMSTRING STRETCH

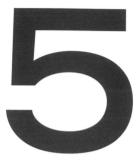

- Lie straight on your back

- Keep your leg as straight as possible and try to gently pull it up until you feel a comfortable stretch. If you need, you can use a towel for help

- Hold for 30 seconds

- Repeat with same side for 3-5 times

- Repeat with other leg

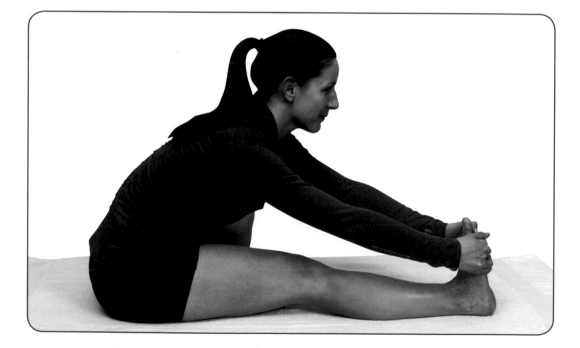

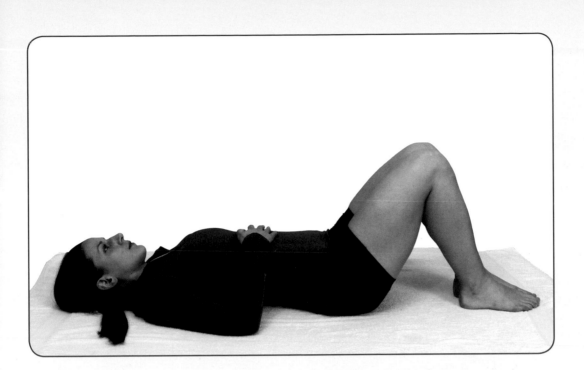

PELVIC LIFT

- Lie on your back, keeping your knees bent and feet flat on the floor

- Now, push down through your feet and slowly lift your bottom up from the floor

- Hold for 10 seconds

- Return to original position and repeat 10 times

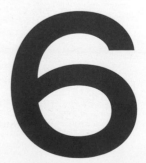

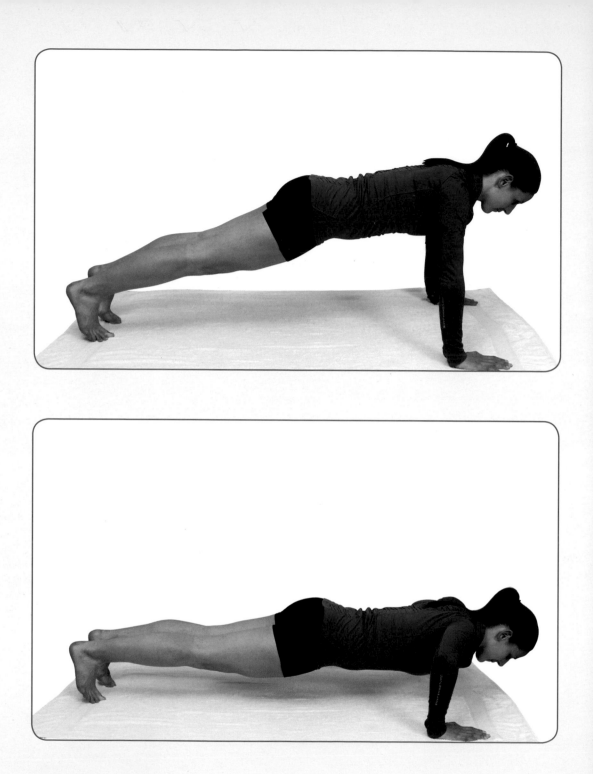

PUSH-UP

- Lie flat on your stomach

- Place your hands and palms down, under your shoulders

- Straighten your arms and raise your upper trunk away from the floor

- Keep your pelvis against the mat and allow your lower back to form an arch

- Hold for 5 seconds

- Return to normal position and repeat

- If push-ups are difficult then bend your knees. Do the push-ups on your knees and not your feet

Note

Each of these exercises should ideally be done at least five times, twice a day, and gradually going up to 10 times, twice a day or as advised by your physiotherapist. Experts warn that you should not push past tolerable levels of pain when you exercise. If you experience pain while performing an exercise then modify your regimen. Either decrease the number of repetitions or reduce the number of sets you do per day. The exercises should be done for 21 days at a stretch. By the third, fourth or fifth day there should be a decrease in the symptoms. Consult your therapist if you see no improvement.

All exercises in this and the following section are advised to be done over a period of 21 days, as it takes as many days to break a habit. By instilling an exercise program that works, you are helping the body to heal in a natural manner.

PRECAUTIONS

Though a regular exercise regimen is advisable for overall fitness, there are certain exercises that could aggravate your suffering if you overdo them. Remember to do the following activities only if you can tolerate the discomfort.

- Football

- Jogging

- Golf

- Weight lifting

- Leg lifts, especially when lying flat on your stomach

- Sit-ups, done with straight legs

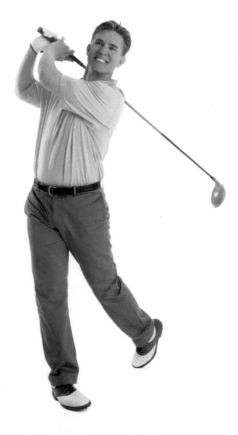

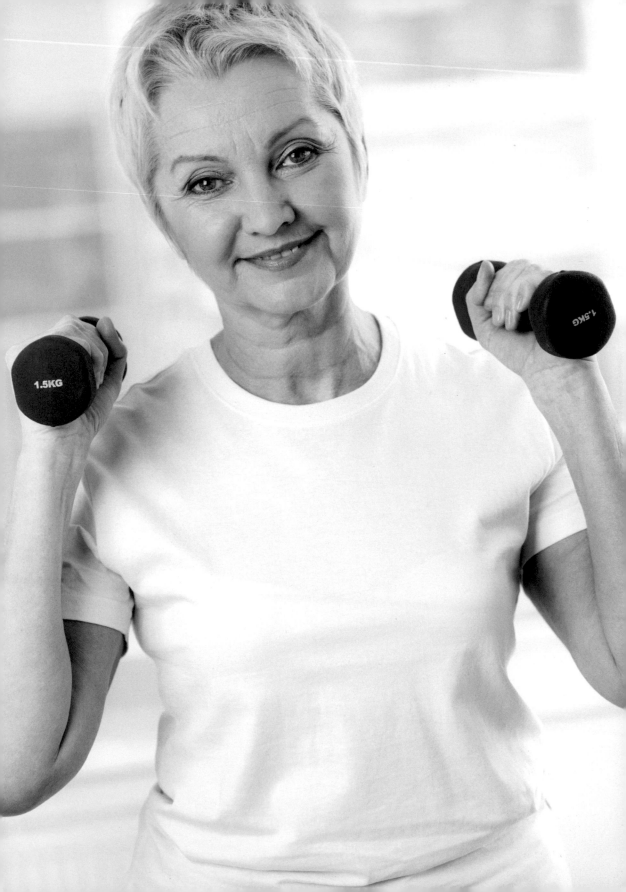

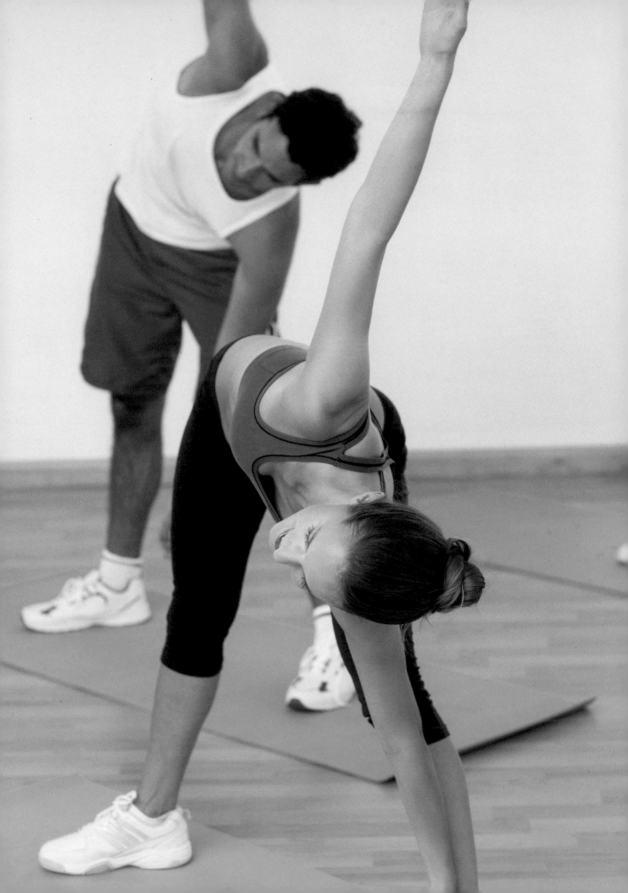

PILATES

Pilates is a comprehensive exercise program that encompasses the entire human body and is known to have a therapeutic effect for low back pain.

"It is the mind itself that shapes the body."
– Joseph Pilates, Founder

How does it work?

Pilates works by focusing on developing the core strength of the body and improving posture through a series of low impact, low repetition stretching and conditioning exercises. It is basically designed to strengthen and restore the human body. Pilates also lays a strong emphasis on breathing and body awareness.

Pilates works on the basis of six core principles, including the following:

- **Centering, bringing the focus of all exercises to the centre of the body**

- **Concentration, promising maximum benefit if the exercises are done with focus and commitment**

- **Control, especially muscle control, which should be present in each exercise**

- **Precision, which should be maintained along with awareness of the positioning and movement of each of the body parts in all the exercises**

- **Breath, the patterns for which are integrated through Pilates exercises**

- **Flow, that needs to be maintained in a smooth manner through each of the exercises**

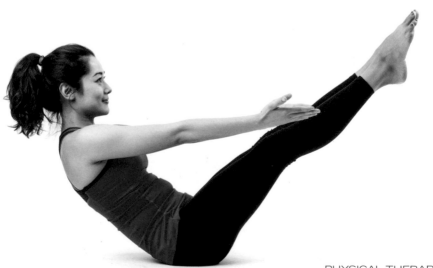

YOGA

Yoga is widely considered as one of the highly effective forms of physical therapies to obtain relief from low back pain. In fact, yoga is known to alleviate the stress associated with low back pain to a great extent, thereby reducing the overall sensation of pain. However, experts recommend following correct instructions and consulting your physician before starting on any yogic exercises as some of the exercises can actually aggravate your condition.

Here I'll briefly explain some of the most helpful yoga exercises you can perform to obtain relief from your low back pain.

Yoga is widely considered
as one of the highly
effective forms of physical
therapies to obtain relief
from low back pain.

THE TOP 5 YOGA WORKOUTS

CORPSE

1

- Lie flat on your back

- Keep your arms resting at your sides, palms down and legs lying naturally

- Maintaining a relaxed position, keep your legs turned out slightly

- Breathe in and out slowly for a few seconds, allowing all waves of tension to escape the body

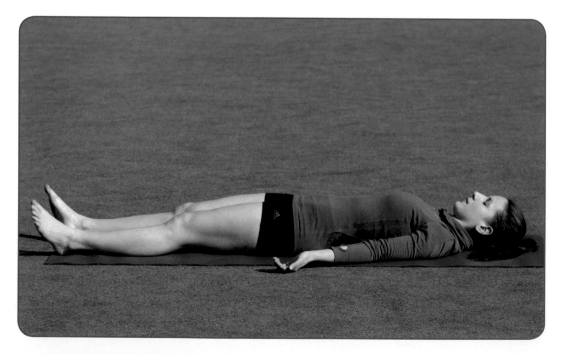

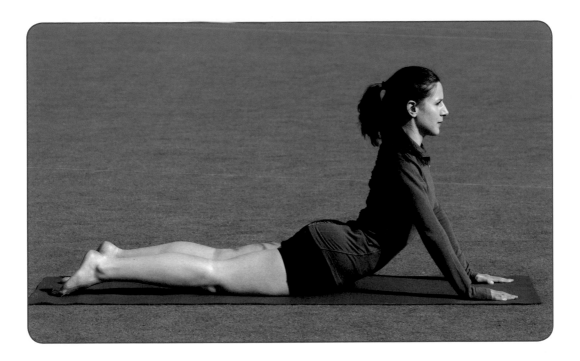

COBRA POSE

- Bring yourself into the prone position

- Place your hands down under the shoulders

- Now try to raise your upper body

- Push the legs together if you can comfortably manage to do so

- In case you want a deeper stretch, you can also leave your legs slightly open

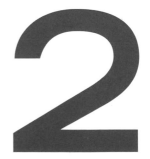

PALM TREE

- Stand with your feet facing forward, arms at your sides and weight distributed on both feet

- Raise your arms over your head and interlock your hands

- Now turn your hands in such a manner that your palms are facing upwards

- Place your palms on the head and turn your head, looking slightly upward

- Now stretch your arms upwards and come up to your toes, if it isn't painful

- Finally, stretch your entire body upward and hold, for 5-8 seconds, depending on your ability

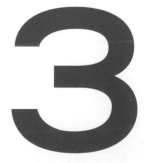

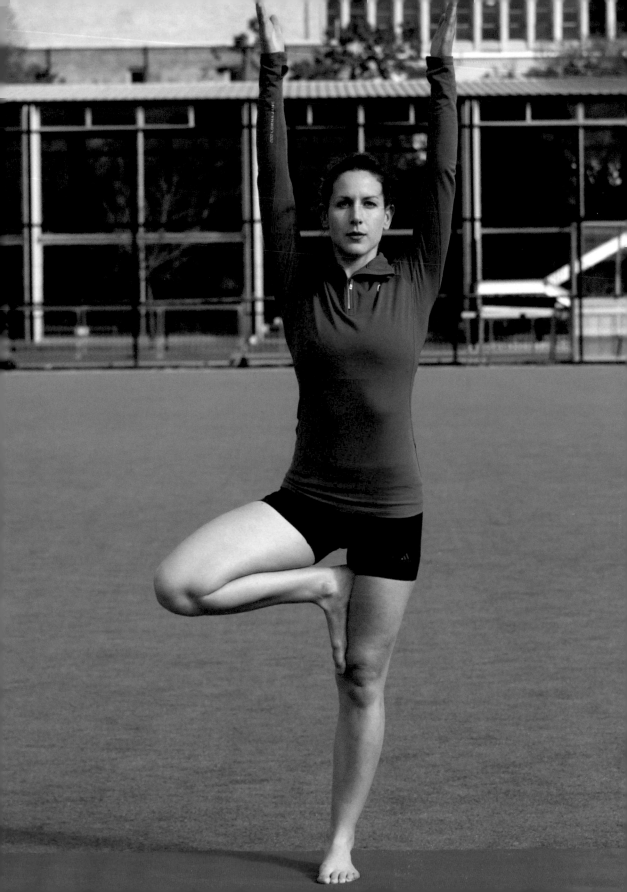

WIND-RELEASING POSE

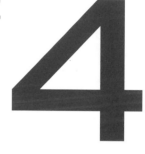

- Lie flat on your back as in the Corpse pose. As you inhale in, bend your knee and place your hands right below your knee

- Draw your legs towards your chest

- Exhale and bring your forehead up to touch your knees

- Inhale again and now exhale as you come to your original position

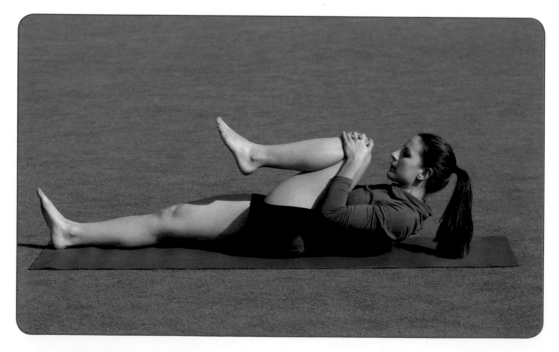

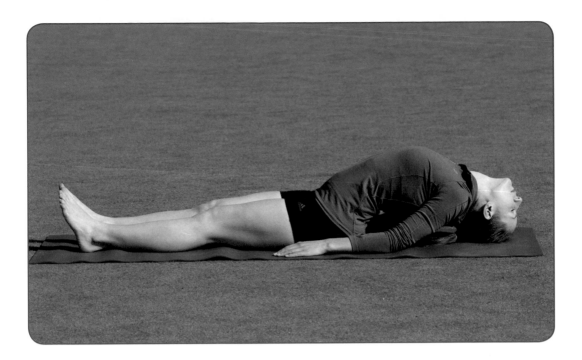

FISH POSE

- Lie on your back, with knees bent and arms at your side

- Try to arch your back until you can do so comfortably and raise it from the ground by pushing the floor with your elbows

- If you can manage to, tilt your head backwards and rest the crown of your head on the floor

- Now, breathe deeply from your diaphragm and hold for maximum one minute, less if you can't manage

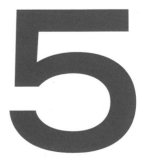

OTHER ACTIVITIES

The listed physical exercises, yogic workouts and Pilates should be further combined with the following forms of activities:

- **Walking**

- **Jogging**

- **Aerobics**

- **Biking**

- **Hydrotherapy**

- **Tai Chi**

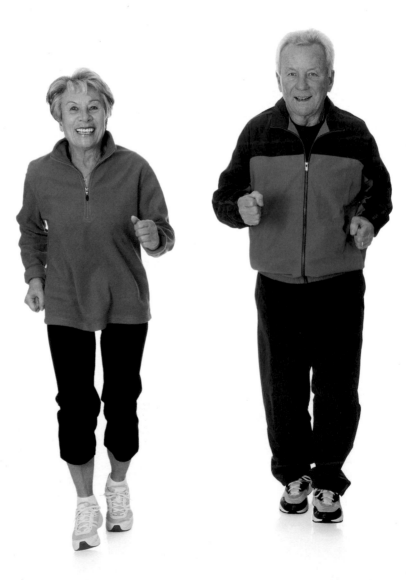

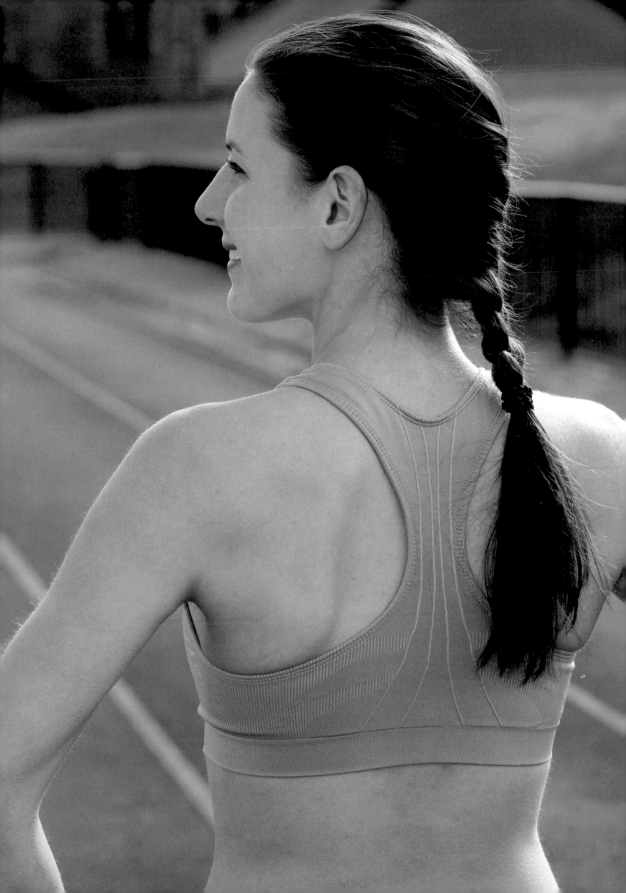

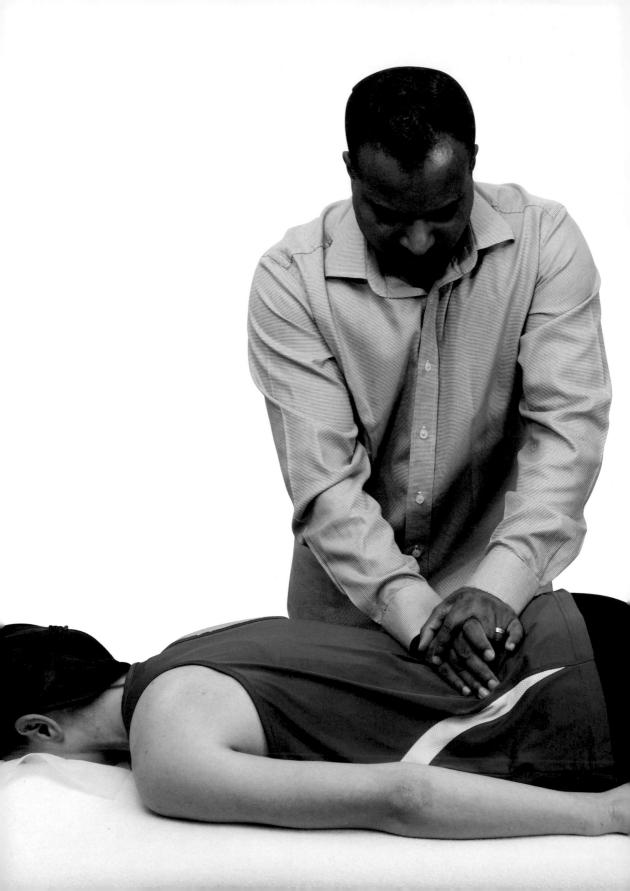

ALTERNATIVE THERAPIES

SPINAL MANIPULATION

Spinal manipulation is one of the most widely studied and accepted forms of alternative therapies for treatment of acute low back pain. This therapy works on the basis of the assumption that a restricted or misaligned spine causes health issues as it hampers the health-maintaining energy flow of the human body.

Experts believe that the human body is capable of healing itself when the spine is aligned and is given the freedom of movement. Viewing the mind and body as twin sides of the same mechanism, this form of treatment pays special attention to the significance of alignment between the spinal cord and the state of health.

How does it work?

There are a number of techniques used for spinal manipulation. To begin with, in order to adjust or realign the spine, physiotherapists use hand movements to apply sudden pressure or force on the spine, trying to extend it beyond the normal range of motion it generally has. Though such treatments are rarely painful, patients might often hear sounds of cracking or popping in the course of the treatment, which is quite normal and should not be a cause of alarm.

As a secondary technique, the physiotherapist might massage or stretch the muscles to bring about the re-alignment of the spine. In some cases, other techniques might also be used to facilitate the spinal re-alignment, including the likes of electrical stimulation, specific exercises, nutrition counselling and heat and ice therapy.

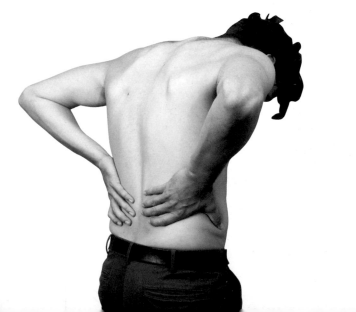

BIOFEEDBACK TECHNIQUES

In this form of alternative therapy, the practitioner teaches the patient the mental as well as physical exercises that are simultaneously monitored by sensors attached to specific points in the body. Each of these sensors is further attached to a machine which is designed to monitor the physiological responses.

HEAT THERAPY

Warmth and heat have always been associated with comfort and pain relief. However, in the case of low back pain, heat therapy offers a twin benefit to the patient i.e. relief from pain and help in healing. To begin with, heat therapy is useful when the cause of low back pain has been ascertained as a strain and overexertion.

Types of Heat Therapy

Dry Heat: In this type of heat therapy, dry heat - such as electric heating pads and saunas - are used to draw out moisture from the body, thus leading to a lot of hydration in the skin.

Moist Heat: The most common source of moist heat is a hot bath, which can facilitate heat's penetration into the muscles considerably.

Common Forms

The most common methods used for heat therapy include:

- **Hot water bottle**

- **Heated gel packs**

- **Heat wraps**

- **Electric heating pad**

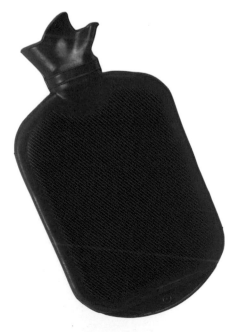

The most common
source of moist heat
is a hot bath, which
can facilitate heat's
penetration into the
muscles considerably.

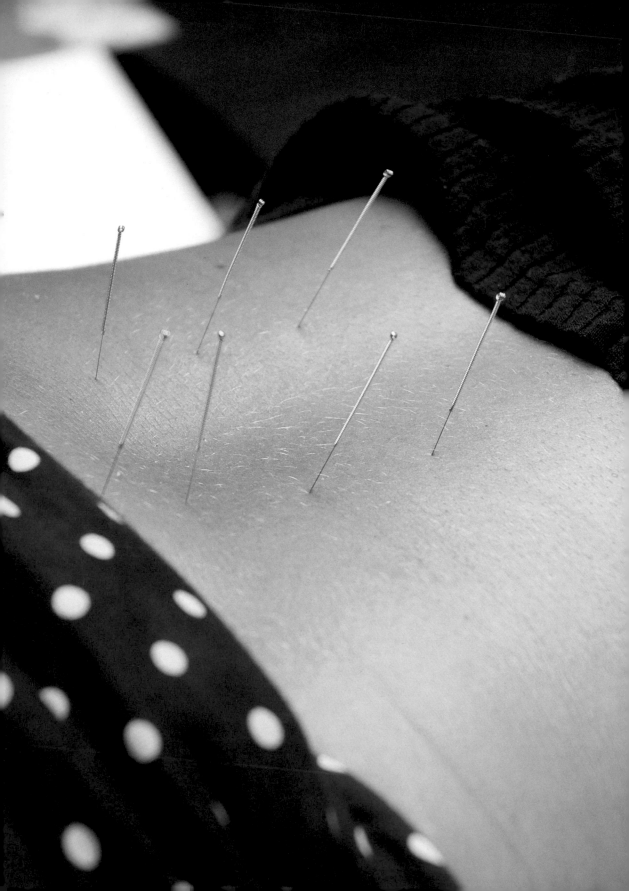

TRANSCUTANEOUS ELECTRICAL NERVE STIMULATION (TENS)

TENS is a form of complementary therapy that relieves back pain by delivering mild electric pulses to the painful area through the electrodes on the skin. These electrodes are further expected to stimulate your nerve fibers, eventually blocking the pain signals to the brain. Low back pain mostly responds well to the TENS therapy, especially when administered in combination with medical treatments.

ALTERNATIVE MEDICINE

In problems such as low back pain, defining a specific cause of the problem usually becomes difficult. In addition, it has often been found that the conventional forms of medication might not have the desired therapeutic effect on low back pain. It is in such circumstances that you might want to look at other alternative forms of treatment.

The modalities of alternative therapy are generally adopted in order to achieve one or more of the following objectives:

- **To relax the tension in muscles**

- **To rectify the spinal imbalances**

- **To relieve discomfort**

- **To ward off risks of long-term problems in the back by improving strength of the muscles and joint stability**

Read on for a detailed insight into how alternative therapies can be of help when you are suffering from low back pain that fails to respond to conventional forms of treatment in a satisfactory manner.

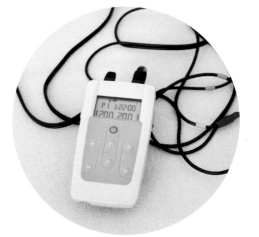

ACUPUNCTURE

If you are not able to gain satisfactory relief from low back pain using conventional forms of treatment then acupuncture might offer substantive relief. Medical research shows acupuncture to be an effective form of treatment of lower back pain, having been successfully studied and used over the last few decades.

Acupuncture attempts to cure by reducing the level of pain and enhancing the overall state of health. Used as part of a comprehensive system of healing known as Oriental Medicine, acupuncture works through the stimulation of certain body points along the meridians and channels that are believed to be the pathways of blood flow in this stream of alternative therapy.

HOMEOPATHY

The use of homeopathic treatments to obtain relief from low back pain has been a subject of research for quite some time. However, there are certain homeopathic remedies that are mostly found effective in the treatment plan for low back pain.

- **Massage and application of Arnica oil to the sore area**

- **Oral doses of Arnica or Rhus toxicodendron**

- **Bellis perennis for deep muscle injuries**

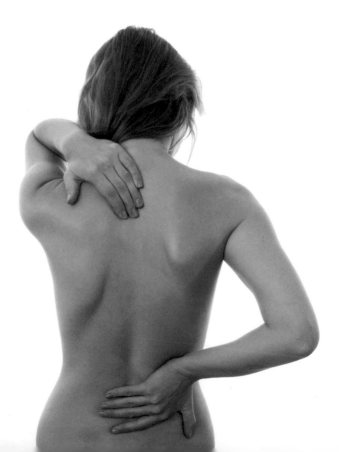

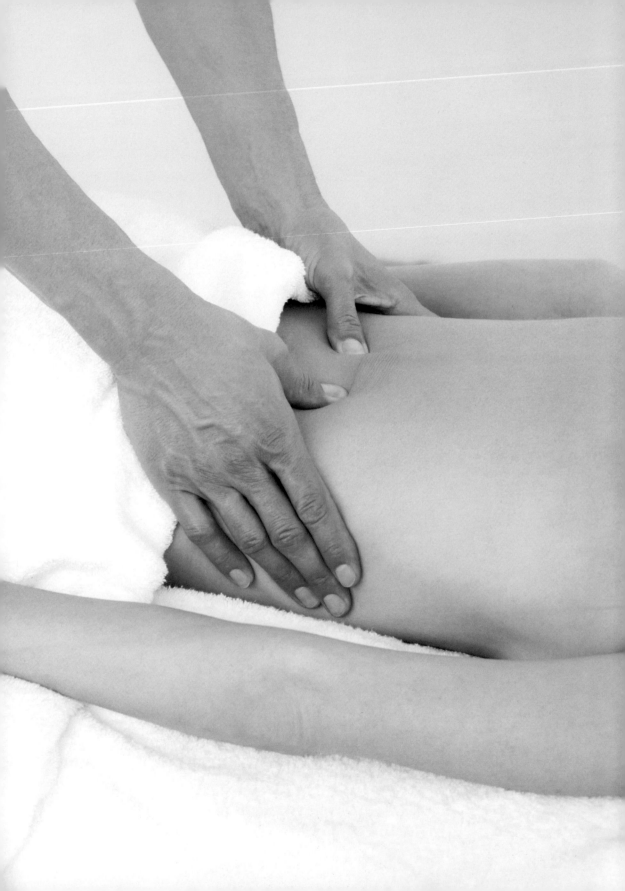

CASE STUDY 5

James, 55 years old

James underwent surgery for his low back pain three years prior to coming into the clinic. He had a laminectomy at the L5/S1 disc level to help alleviate years of pain. James had been a driver for more than 20 years. Years of driving more than 6-8 hours per day had taken its toll. Since the surgery things had improved remarkably but only to about 70%. Obtaining the final 30% would mean that he would have less stiffness, sit for longer than 45 minutes in an arm chair and be able to carry his young granddaughter without apprehension.

Treatment – This constituted a regular routine of physiotherapy sessions, in the first month, where he received eight sessions. He was set up with a hydrotherapy program whereby he exercised in chest level water that was heated to 32 degrees Celsius (Nearly 90 degrees Fahrenheit). The higher temperature meant that the water was very comfortable to be in. When the water level is at chest height a person literally weighs only 25% of their body weight. So someone who weighs 100kg (220lbs) will only weigh 25kg (55lbs) at that depth. This makes exercising more tolerable, lifts the load on muscles and joints that are more load bearing (lower back, hips, knees and ankles). James completed a 12-week hydrotherapy program, which he attended twice a week (45 minutes per session). This addressed his core and also his functional control. This allowed him to sit for longer than 1 hour (he liked watching movies) and carry his granddaughter with more ease.

This constituted a regular routine of physiotherapy sessions, in the first month, where he received eight sessions

CASE STUDY 6

Jenny, 7 years old

Jenny had been dancing since the age of three. She loved ballet but the rigorous daily training sessions were becoming more intensive. Her flexibility was decreasing and this was affecting her performances.

Treatment – Jenny's biomechanics were impeded by her core not catching up to her rigorous training schedules. A 12 week supervised Pilates program was introduced. These were one-on-one sessions with a therapist. Each session saw her test her core out with added intensity. This graduated program meant that she could tolerate more loading from her training. She was also given a 15 minute per day Pilates home exercise program, which she did religiously. After 12 weeks of core control training Jenny made a full recovery. She does come in for a tune up every two to four weeks when she is performing. During the off season her tune ups are stretched out to every three to six months.

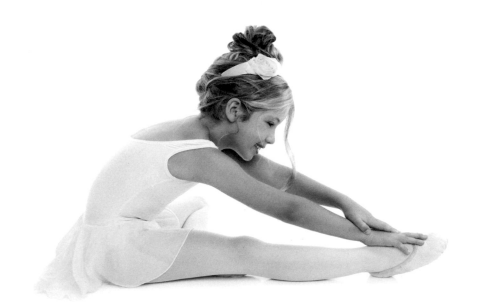

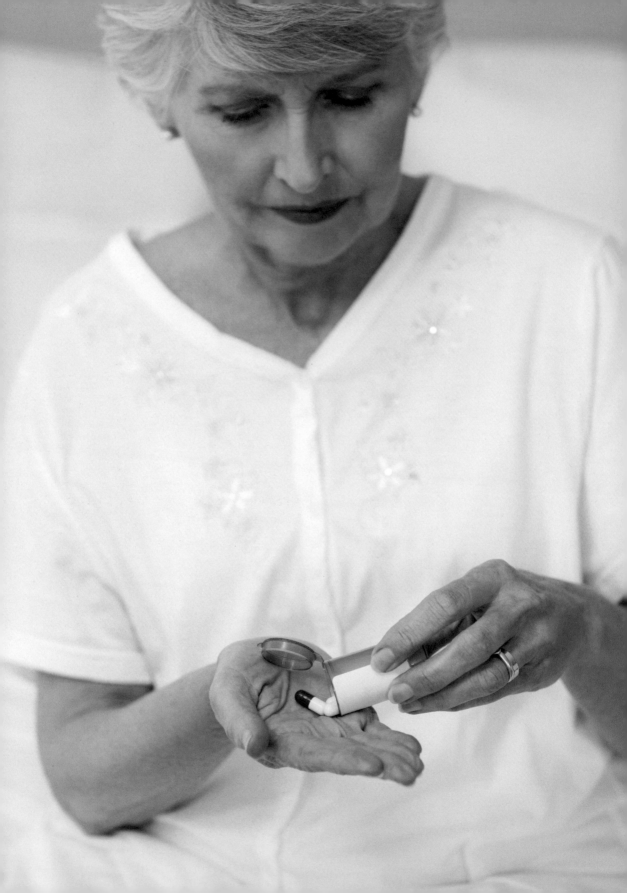

MEDICAL TREATMENT

CONVENTIONAL MEDICINE

Conventional medicine refers to the cluster of medications most commonly used to obtain relief from human disorders. Conventional medicines have been found to be one of the most effective forms of treatments available for low back pain. However, as is the case for all medications, medicines prescribed for low back pain also have their own side effects, which can vary.

Read on for detailed information on various medications prescribed for low back pain and their possible side effects, if any, along with any other important facts the patient needs to know.

PAINKILLERS

. . . .

Painkillers used for obtaining relief form LBP are usually divided into two broad categories, including the over-the-counter (OTC) drugs and the stronger medications.

Over-the-Counter Medications

Some of the most common OTC medications prescribed for low back pain include:

- **Paracetamol (Panadol)**

- **Ibuprofen (Advil)**

- **Naproxen (Naprosyn)**

- **Aspirin**

The above listed OTC drugs are usually safe and can be administered without consulting a medical professional. These are usually considered as the first form of medication given for LBP, especially the one lasting for a short period of time.

However, the use of OTC drugs is not recommended for individuals suffering from the following conditions, unless advised otherwise:

- **Bleeding**

- **Heart problems**

- **Kidney disorder**

- **Liver problems**

Prescription Drugs

Stronger medications advised for relief from low back pain include the prescription strength NSAIDs, such as ibuprofen and naproxen. However, opioids are considered to be the strongest form of pain-relieving medication and need to be administered under strict medical supervision, and only for patients with acute pain. The use of opioids is also accompanied by a strong possibility of side effects, including the following:

- **Constipation**

- **Nausea**

- **Sleepiness**

In some cases, opioids can also lead to addiction and severe substance abuse.

MUSCLE RELAXANTS

Muscle relaxants are generally used as a secondary option to pain relieving medications and are quite useful, especially when taken before bedtime, though mostly for shorter durations. Such skeletal muscle relaxants are known to alleviate pain and improve functional ability. However, most muscle relaxants come with the possibility of drowsiness and should be administered with care.

ANTIDEPRESSANTS

Antidepressants, especially tricyclic antidepressants have been found to be moderately effective as a medication for low back pain. Since depression and anxiety are believed to be generally present in patients with low back pain, this class of medication is believed to be quite effective in alleviating such symptoms. Most common drugs used in this category include:

- **Amitriptyline**

- **Nortriptyline**

- **Desipramine**

- **Venlafaxine**

- **Duloxetine**

Other medications such as Gabapentin and corticosteroids have also been found to be effective in curing low back pain, though results vary.

Antidepressants, especially tricyclic antidepressants have been found to be moderately effective as a medication for low back pain.

SPINAL INJECTIONS

Spinal injections are quite commonly used as a treatment for low back pain. Such injections are administered with two key objectives in sight, including:

- **To alleviate pain**

- **To serve as a diagnostic tool, helping to ascertain the cause of pain**

There are two forms of spinal injections that are commonly used for relief from low back pain, including the following:

Facet Joint Injections

The facet joint injection aims to decrease inflammation and pain that arises from one or more of the facet joints. Located at the back of the spine, the facet joints are extremely important for movement and mobility.

Epidural Steroid Injections

The epidural steroid injections work by injecting pain relieving medications into the epidural spaces. Once administered, the medicine flows through the epidural space, coating nerve roots along with the outside lining of the facet joints.

In addition to the above, there are other injections that are administered into the muscles, soft tissues and the regions of the deeper back for gaining relief from low back pain. The most common injections amongst these include:

- **Trigger point injections, in which a local anesthetic is administered into the superficial muscles or soft tissues**

- **Chemonucleolysis, in which an enzyme is injected into a herniated disc in order to shrink the disc and relieve pressure on a compressed nerve root**

- **Prolotherapy, involving an injection of irritant chemicals into soft tissues of the back**

SURGICAL INTERVENTION

Surgical procedures are mostly resorted to as the last option for low back pain. In severe low back conditions, spinal surgery becomes important to relieve the pressure on nerves or alleviate pain in general.

In the following section, I'll briefly discuss the main types of back surgeries that can offer relief from low back pain.

Spinal Discectomy

A discectomy is performed for the treatment of herniated discs. This procedure involves removal of the soft gel-like material that gets herniated out of the disc, compressing a spinal nerve. Discectomy is typically aimed at returning the disc to a better and more normal shape. It also aims to relieve the pressure on the spinal nerve located nearby.

FORAMENOTOMY

Foramenotomy is also a back surgery used to relieve the pressure on nerves like discectomy. However, in foramenotomy the nerve is actually being pinched by reasons other than a herniated disc. Hence, foramenotomy cures the problem by removing a portion of the bone and other related tissue which might be compressing the nerve.

LAMINECTOMY

This particular procedure is carried out in order to relieve pressure that is being exerted on the spinal cord. Most common conditions that get treated using a laminectomy include spinal stenosis and spondylolisthesis. At times, this particular procedure is done along with spinal fusion to prevent any scope of instability.

Spinal Fusion

Spinal fusion is a surgery that is carried out to link two or more vertebrae together. Low back pain is often caused due to a problem with the disc space, which can be effectively treated with spine fusion. This form of surgery aims to remove the movement that occurs within the effected portion of the spine, thereby striving to eliminate the basic cause of low back pain.

This type of procedure usually involves instrumentation, which includes use of medical devices such as cages, plates, screws and rods as well as bone grafts in order to stabilise the spine. The bone graft materials used generally include:

- **Patient's own graft (autograft)**

- **Donor bone (allograft)**

- **Bone morphogenetic protein (BMP)**

Spinal Disc Replacement Surgery

Having been recently approved in the USA as an acceptable form of treatment for some types of low back pain, the spinal disc replacement surgery is becoming one of the most result-oriented forms of LBP treatments.

In this type of surgery, the biological disc or the degenerated disc material is removed. Once done, an artificial intervertebral disc is implanted in the spine. It also helps to know that the disc replacement surgery is normally much less invasive than the traditional spinal surgery. In fact, the recovery time associated with this type of surgery is usually less than the other forms, such as spine fusion.

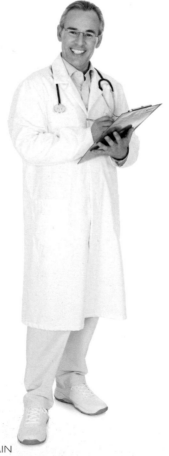

MEDICAL PROFESSIONALS

A series of medical professionals normally need to be involved in a typical treatment plan for low back pain. Most commonly included medical professionals are:

- **Orthopedic surgeons**

- **Physiotherapists**

- **Occupational therapists**

- **Surgical specialists**

- **Psychologists**

- **Nurses**

DIAGNOSIS

The formulation of a result-oriented and effective treatment plan for low back pain depends largely on the diagnosis of the condition and the probable cause of the pain.

A scientifically designed diagnostic plan for low back pain usually comprises of three steps, including:

1 **Understanding patient history**

2 **Physical examination**

3 **Imaging procedures**

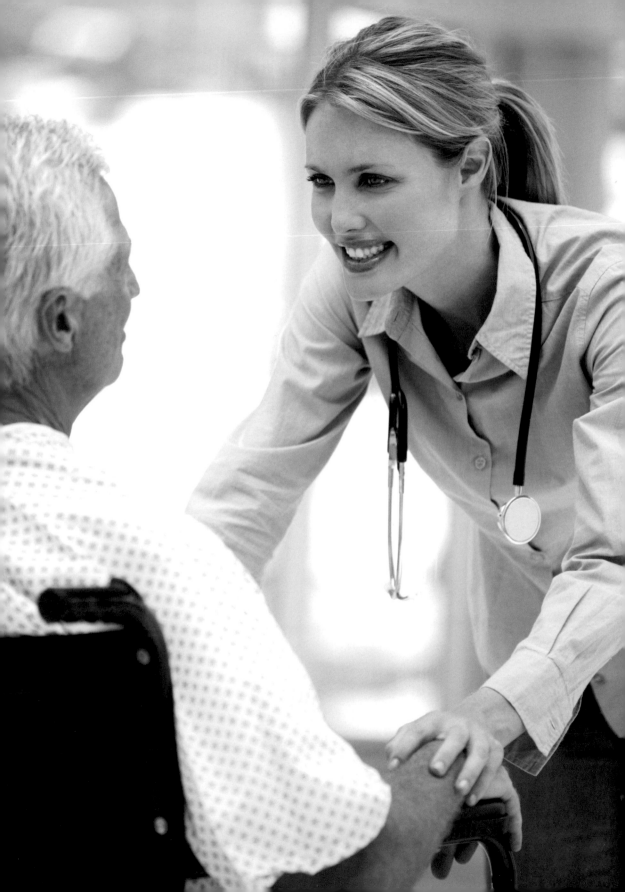

The physical examination of the patient is done with the specific objective to locate the source of pain and determine the limits of movement caused by it.

Patient History

To begin with, the physician needs an insight into your medical history. This is important for the physician to be able to determine any correlation between the current LBP episode and any previous medical history. Various aspects of medical history and information that needs to be noted and examined include:

- **Any background or history of heart problems, cancer or arthritis in the family of the patient**

- **Any history of accidents or injuries that involve the neck, back or hips**

- **Any signs of conditions like excessive unexplained weight loss or chronic infection**

- **Any instances where normal activities like coughing, sneezing, exercising or walking aggravate the problem**

- **Any specific activity that might provide respite from the pain, such as lying or sitting down or exercising**

- **Any previous episodes of back pain**

- **Pattern of frequency and duration of the pain**

- **Any specific pattern of the timing of back pain**

- **Any specific problems related to bowel or bladder control**

- **Any other specific symptoms like morning stiffness, numbness or weakness in legs**

Physical Examination

The physical examination of the patient is done with the specific objective to locate the source of pain and determine the limits of movement caused by it.

In most of the cases, the patient is asked to perform certain activities and movements that will help diagnose the exact cause and location of pain.

MAIN ACTIVITIES

- **Sit, stand or walk in different ways. These include flat-footed, on the toes, on the heels etc**

- **Bend forwards, backwards, sideways and twist**

- **Lift your leg straight up while lying down**

- **Observe circumference of the calves and thighs that will help in determining any presence of muscle deterioration**

In addition to the above, the physician might also conduct special tests to examine the integrity of nerve functions and reflexes.

Imaging Procedures

In order to point out the exact cause of low back pain, a series of imaging procedures are carried out. The exact types of imaging studies carried out depend upon the specific signs being shown by the patient and the severity of symptoms. In case the patient is not suffering from a single underlying cause, a combination of diagnostic methods might need to be applied. Here I've listed brief definitions of various kinds of imaging tools used for diagnosis of low back pain.

1 **X-Rays: This is the most common method that helps in detecting the cause and location of back pain and uses basic imaging technique**

2 **Magnetic Resonance Imaging (MRI): This can be used to examine the lumbar region and provides a three-dimensional view of the area. Unlike an X-ray it does not expose the patient to radiation**

3 **Computerised Tomography (CT): This is a painless procedure that is used when damage to the vertebrae is suspected to be a cause of low back pain**

4 **Discography: This involves the injection of a contrast dye into the spinal disc that is suspected to be the cause of low back pain**

5 **Magnetic Resonance Imaging (MRI): This is used to examine the lumbar region**

6 **Electrodiagnostic procedures: This includes electromyography (EMG), nerve conductions studies and evoked potential (EP) studies**

7 **Bone scans: These are used to diagnose and monitor infections, disorders in the bone and fractures**

8 **Thermography: This imaging method uses infrared sensing devices to measure small temperature alterations**

9 **Ultrasound imaging: This procedure uses high-frequency sound waves to obtain images inside the human body**

PROGNOSIS

Research shows the prognosis to be effective in most of the cases of low back pain. As many as 80% of the patients are reported to recover completely in a time span of 4-6 weeks. Meanwhile, the prognosis for patients suffering from chronic pain depends on the actual underlying cause of the pain.

Most often, the effective treatment of low back pain emanates from a combination of treatments in specific context to the patient's medical history and current symptoms. For instance, one particular patient suffering from LBP might benefit from a combination of massage and medications, while another might get relief from a combination of medications and exercise.

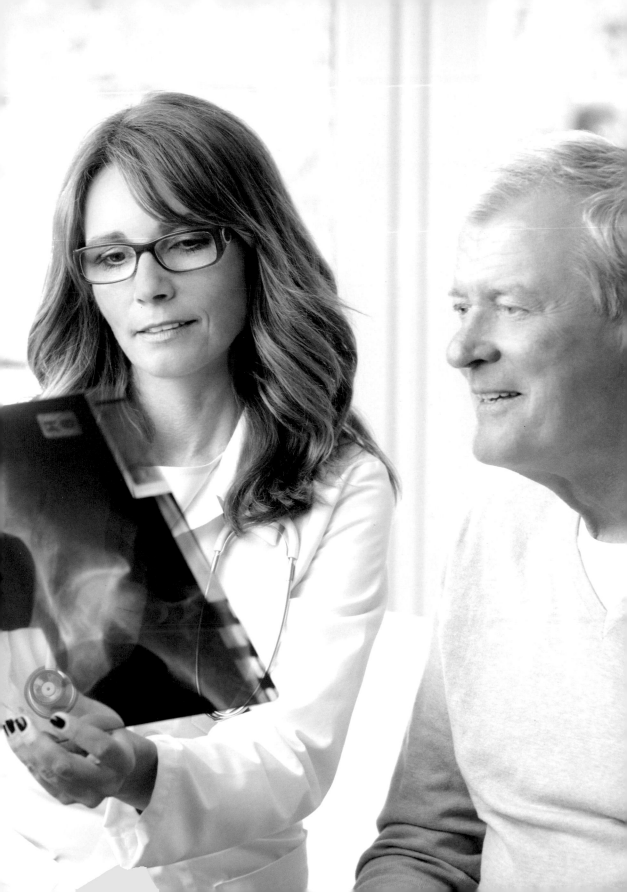

CASE STUDY 7

Anna, 11 years old

Anna was going through a growth spurt. Many children suffer from spinal pain, knee pain and joint pain when going through growth spurts. Anna's pain was primarily in her back. Her bones were growing faster than her muscles. When there is a discrepancy between these two structures pain results.

Also girls at this age are more self conscious – they are growing taller and usually become taller than the boys in their classes. This causes them to hunch more or round their shoulders further.

Treatment – Anna was treated for four sessions by her physiotherapist who improved her alignment, educated her in the importance of spinal posture and taught her an exercise program to help keep the muscles in control until the growth spurt ended. The exercise program included swimming and cycling, both low weight bearing activities that kept the muscles working but active. She would do two sessions of swimming or cycling (60 minutes per session) each week. Her pain was under control and she was pain free in four weeks. Every three months she comes in for a tune up with her physiotherapist to make sure her alignment and the underlying causative factors are monitored.

The exercise program included swimming and cycling, both low weight bearing activities that kept the muscles working but active

CASE STUDY 8

Martina, 28 years old

Martina is an office worker who started getting a stiff back two months prior to treatment. She was getting busier at work but no amount of treatment by previous therapists would help her be pain free. Treatment to help her biomechanics, range, control, core and strength would only help so much. She had improved to about 75% during sessions but every morning when she awoke she would feel stiff – the gains from the previous day seemed lost.

Treatment – Martina's bed was more than 10 years old. The springs of the mattress had now worn and the ideal support she was supposed to get with eight hours of sleep wasn't occurring. This lack of support meant all the hard work her therapists had achieved was lost. Martina trialled sleeping in a different room in her house (that had a newer mattress). Even after one night she woke up feeling fresher, with no discomfort, and the gains from her previous treatment had 'stuck'. She then bought a new mattress.

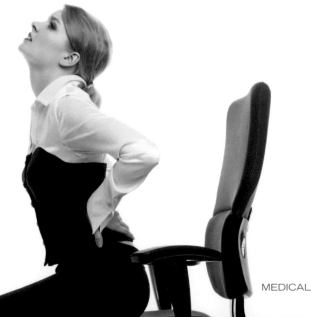

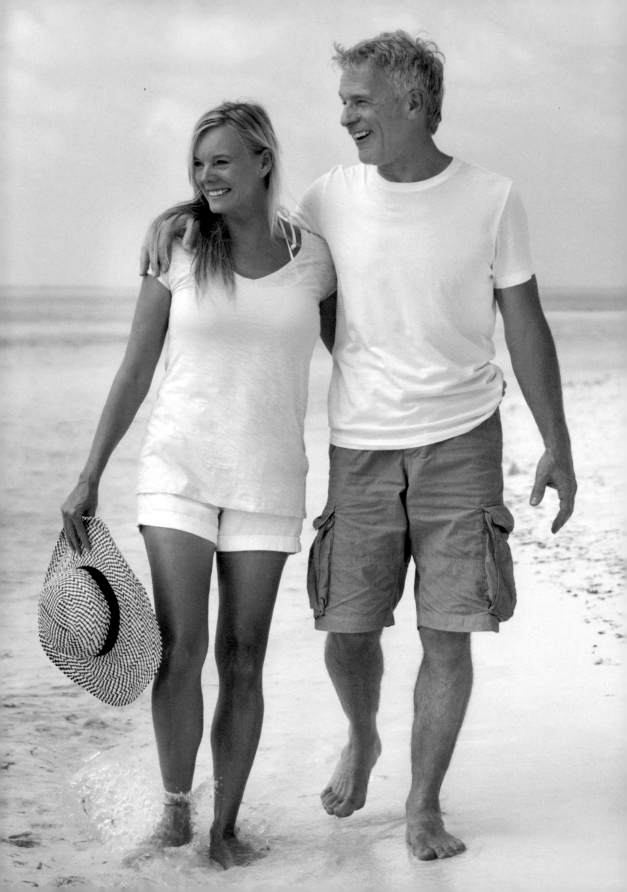

THE LATEST DEVELOPMENTS IN BACK PAIN – THE PERFORMANCE PYRAMID

There are five fundamentals in the body that need to be fulfilled so it works at an optimum level. This means that when the five fundamentals are achieved there is no pain, no discomfort, no apprehension with movement, and no stiffness.

After 50,000 treatments over a 15 year period these key fundamentals were identified because they brought the best results in the shortest period of time for back pain sufferers.

These are the five fundamentals:

BIOMECHANICS

. . . .

The Biomechanics in the body constitute the nerves, muscles, joints and ligaments in the body. Their analysis involves how they interact with a person's movement, activities they conduct in their everyday life, and their involvement in a person's behaviour. For example stress can affect how the biomechanics function therefore affecting a person's functional ability. The Biomechanics fundamental is the most important fundamental and is the foundation of the pyramid.

FUNCTIONAL RANGE

Once the foundation is set a person should be able to move. This is their range. Range allows the person to bend forwards and backwards. If the biomechanics weren't functioning well then a person's functional range would be poor. This is the second most important fundamental.

FUNCTIONAL CONTROL

The functional control is the quality of movement. This is crucial for smoothness of movement – the quality of movement. If a person can bend forwards and touch their knees but their movement is 'staggered' or 'step-like' then they are lacking the quality of movement. This lack of quality means that the person's functional control is not optimum. Once the elements in the person's body are good (Biomechanics), and the person achieves their range (Functional Range) then the quality of movement should be improved to guarantee ease of movement (Functional Control).

FUNCTIONAL CORE

A functional core is a stable base. The diaphragm, pelvic floor and a corset-like muscle called the transversus abdominis, work together to provide this stability with movement. If the first three fundamentals are achieved then getting the core correct is next in line.

STRENGTH AND CONDITIONING

This is the final fundamental. This is the cream on the cake. This completes the Pyramid. Strength and Conditioning is vital to maintain the previous fundamentals.

This is the Performance Pyramid that I use and it was created to help back pain sufferers understand which fundamentals weren't performing well and which fundamentals needed 'tweaking'. By breaking down the problem into which fundamentals need 'fixing' a low back pain sufferer can evaluate how much they can do themselves and when they need to see a practitioner. It can also be used to show another practitioner, who they do not see as often, what areas need addressing.

The Performance Pyramid also provides a illustration of the issue. Human beings are creatures who enjoy understanding things in a visual format. If a person understands their issue it is easier find ways to overcome it.

THE ELITE AKADEMY PERFORMANCE PYRAMID

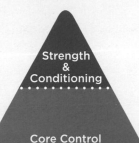

Strength & Conditioning

Core Control

Functional Control

Functional Range

Biomechanics

WEIGHTING SCORE

Strength & Conditioning **4.0**

Core Control **12.0**

Functional Control **20.0**

Functional Range **28.0**

Biomechanics **36.0**

As seen in the diagram on page 107 each element has its weighting.

Biomechanics – 36.0
Functional Range – 28.0
Functional Control – 20.0
Functional Core – 12.0
Strength & Conditioning – 4.0

This outlines the importance of each Fundamental. As you can see the Biomechanics are nine times more important than the Strength and Conditioning Fundamental. Functional Range is seven times more important than Strength and Conditioning, and so on.

This gives sufferers a clear idea on how a rehabilitation process would work. When a person suffers from pain many would say, "I need to get my back stronger", or "I need to work on my core". As the Performance Pyramid shows, many people only concentrate on the top two tiers. This constitutes a total of only 16.0 points of their problem. Many become disheartened and think that they have to live with the pain. The Performance Pyramid allows them to see clearly that there are three more tiers (that add up to 84.0) to achieve before they are feeling better.

Some interesting facts about the Performance Pyramid

For a person to feel comfortable, with no back pain, they would have a total of 85.0 to 95.0. That is, each fundamental is working at 85-95% to achieve this.

If a person scores between 82-85% they will experience apprehension and associated stiffness in their back. If a person scores between 79-81% they will experience pain and stiffness of movement e.g. reluctance to move freely when getting something from the ground. Anything below 78% is pain, stiffness and apprehension.

The most important fundamental – The Biomechanics – have to be evaluated fully by a professional who is experienced in assessing the condition of nerves, muscles, joints and ligaments. To date the most comprehensive practitioners doing this are those who follow the Ridgway Method. This is one of the most up to date clinical reasoning processes in the world today that helps combat pain.

Once the biomechanics are evaluated the person can note which elements in their body need regular tune-ups e.g. the tight joints in the back, gluteal tightness or shoulder issues etc.

The most common mistakes people make in evaluating their Performance Pyramid:

1 They ignore the Biomechanics or they get a non-professional to assess this.

2 They skip steps e.g. they don't address the Functional Range or they ignore the Functional Core fundamental.

3 They are impatient to progress so they push through without reaching an 85% score at each fundamental. This will send them backwards.

Note: it takes approximately 4-12 weeks to work through the fundamentals.

The diagram below shows how each element can be scored. (EA PP Scoring) This scoring system was devised to provide feedback to the pain sufferer and to bring awareness to how much work was needed for them to feel better. Each fundamental can also be assessed, and this is usually done by a professional. However, to simply understand the five fundamentals can bring enough awareness to most to help self evaluate what is required to solve their back pain.

FUNDAMENTAL	%	YOUR PERFORMANCE SCORE	NORMAL VALUES
Biomechanics 36.0			30.6 – 34.2
Functional Range 28.0			23.8 – 26.6
Functional Control 20.0			17.0 – 19.0
Functional Core 12.0			10.2 – 11.4
Strength & Conditioning 4.0			3.4 – 3.8
		Your Peak Performance Score	Peak Performance 85.0 – 95.0

THE LAST WORD

Patient participation is crucial to the success of a treatment program for low back pain. Intimidating as it might sound, low back pain is surely within the realms of treatment and cure, especially if detected at an early stage. Right decisions taken in time and reported to medical professionals can save you a lifetime of pain and misery, not to mention the loss of efficiency you might have to face due to your nagging pain.

Get set and educate yourself about your symptoms, causes and the treatment choices available to you. The cure and relief is for you to ask for. Science has surely left no stone unturned to devise result-oriented treatment modalities and it's time you, as a learned individual, begin to seek maximum benefits from such blissful gifts of the modern life.

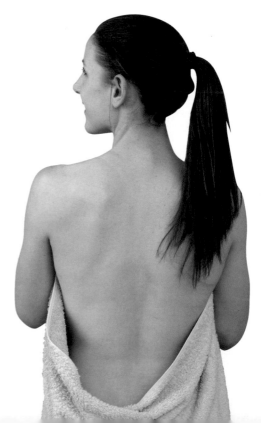

BACK PAIN JOURNAL

	QUESTIONS TO ASK YOURSELF	TICK ON THE APPROPRIATE CHOICE		
1	On which side do you feel the LBP most often?	Left	Right	Both
2	How do you classify your LBP?	Dull	Sharp	Burning
3	Have you suffered from LBP before?	Yes	No	
4	How did the LBP start?	Suddenly	Gradually	
5	Have you suffered from any of these?	Injury	Accident	Neither
6	Were you doing any of these activities before LBP started?	Lifting/ Bending	Working on the computer	Driving for long hours
7	Is your current LBP different from any previous episode of LBP you've had?	Yes	No	No LBP earlier
8	Are you aware of the causes of the previous episodes of LBP?	Yes	No	No LBP earlier
9	How long is each episode of LBP?	30 minutes – 1 hour	1 hour – 5 hours	More than 5 hours
10	Apart from LBP, do you feel pain in any of these parts?	Hip/Thigh	Leg/Feet	
11	Apart from LBP, do you have any of the following?	Numbness/ Tingling	Loss of function in any other part of body?	Weakness
12	Do long periods of any of these activities aggravate your LBP?	Lifting/ Twisting	Standing/ Sitting	
13	Which therapy makes you feel better?	Medicines	Exercise	Any other
14	Are you experiencing any of these symptoms?	Weight loss	Fever	Change in urination/ bowel habits

INDEX

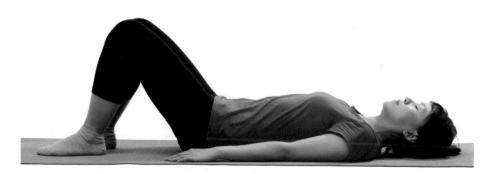